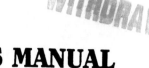
THERAPY OUTCOME MEASURES MANUAL
Physiotherapy, Occupational Therapy, Rehabilitation Nursing

THERAPY OUTCOME MEASURES MANUAL
Physiotherapy, Occupational Therapy, Rehabilitation Nursing

Professor Pam Enderby Ph.D., M.Sc., F.C.S.L.T., M.B.E.

with

Alexandra John M.Sc., DipCST

and

Brian Petheram, BA, PhD

The University of Sheffield
Community Sciences Center
Northern General Hospital
Sheffield, England

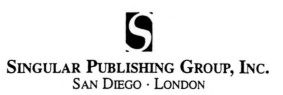

SINGULAR PUBLISHING GROUP, INC.
SAN DIEGO · LONDON

Singular Publishing Group, Inc.
401 West "A" Street, Suite 325
San Diego, California 92101-7904

Singular Publishing Group Ltd.
19 Compton Terrace
London, N1 2UN, UK

Singular Publishing Group, Inc., publishes textbooks, clinical manuals, clinical reference books, journals, videos, and multimedia materials on speech-language pathology, audiology, otorhinolaryngology, special education, early childhood, aging, occupational therapy, physical therapy, rehabilitation, counseling, mental health, and voice. For your convenience, our entire catalog can be accessed on our website at *http://www.singpub.com*. Our mission to provide you with materials to meet the daily challenges of the ever-changing health care/educational environment will remain on course if we are in touch with you. In that spirit, we welcome your feedback on our products. Please telephone (**1-800-521-8545**), fax (**1-800-774-8398**), or e-mail (*singpub@mail.cerfnet.com*) your comments and requests to us.

Typeset in 12/15 Palatino by So Cal Graphics

Library of Congress Cataloging-in-Publication Data

Enderby, Pamela M. (Pamela Mary), 1949–
    Therapy outcome measures manual: physiotherapy, occupational therapy, rehabilitation nursing/Pam Enderby; with Alexandra John and Brian Petheram.
       p.   cm.
   ISBN 1-56593-995-6
    1. Medical rehabilitation. 2. Outcome assessment (Medical care).
I. John, Alexandra. II. Petheram, Brian. III. Title.
    [DNLM: 1. Physical Therapy—methods handbooks. 2. Outcome
Assessment (Health Care)—methods handbooks. 3. Disability
Evaluation handbooks. 4. Occupational Therapy—methods handbooks.
5. Rehabilitation Nursing—methods handbooks. WB 39 E57t 1998]
RM930.E53 1998
615.8'2—dc21
DNLM/DLC
for Library of Congress
                                                       98-17801
                                                        CIP

CONTENTS

PREFACE

The therapy outcome measure (TOM) allows therapists to describe the relative abilities/difficulties of a patient in the four domains of impairment, disability, handicap and well-being in order to monitor changes over time. This approach, which has been rigorously tested for reliability and clinical validity, can be used by physiotherapists, occupational therapists, rehabilitation nurses and speech and language therapists (separate manual available). It aims to be quick and simple to use, taking just a few minutes to complete and allows for the aggregation of data so that comparisons can be made. The approach has been trialed in order to establish the differential outcomes between different client groups and different rehabilitation units.

ACKNOWLEDGMENT

A project of this complexity can only be successfully completed if a number of people work consistently and persistently together. Alex and I are grateful for the help we have received from large numbers of physiotherapists, occupational therapists, and nurses who have assisted with the development of the scales, been involved in the reliability studies, and contributed to the data collection. Much of this work was well above and beyond the call of duty!

We thank Lyn Sockett who has patiently redrafted the scales and text and interpreted our unclear requests with telepathic insight.

Gillian Armstrong has directed the statistical analysis of the reliability studies with great fortitude—Thank you.

Pam Enderby

CHAPTER 1

Introduction

Over the last decade there has been an increasing awareness of the importance of being able to gather information to assist in identifying specific gains associated with interventions. There are increasing demands for health care professionals to develop tools to enable them to monitor the progress of patients undergoing treatment.

The pressures on health care investment in all developed countries has been brought about largely by the increasingly ageing population, improvement in health technologies, and the expansion of health interventions along with the greater expectations of society. Purchasers of health care have become alarmed at the apparently inexorable exponential increase in health care costs leading to demands that evidence of effective practice should be required in order to ensure equitable health care provision. Although it is regrettable that health care professionals have taken a particular interest in the effects of their interventions when their programs of work are financially challenged, any stimulus that encourages clinical reflection should be welcomed. Although it is unlikely that outcome measurement and evidence based practice will solve the issues with regard to rationalizing health care costs alone, they may well, inadvertently but fortuitously, have a significant impact on the quality of health care provision.

Over the last two decades there has been an increasing desire by all those in the therapy professions to identify and describe patients' disorders more accurately. This desire has led to a plethora of assessments, many of which are appropriately standardized and validated. These assessments have frequently been used to assist with diagnosis and treatment planning. Less frequently they have been used to monitor change in patients' behavior over time. Thus we enter the new millennium with little objective data about the general progress of the majority of patients through health care programs.

Assessments used by therapists and other health care professionals do not necessarily lend themselves as appropriate tools for outcome measurement. Assessments are very frequently designed to detect, in a sensitive and specific fashion, aspects of a particular disorder for diagnostic purposes. They are often lengthy, not only to administer, but also to analyze, and their focus is commonly on aspects of the impairment or pathological dysfunction.

Outcome measures are needed for different purposes: they should be simple and easy to use, allowing information to be collected on the majority of clients receiving an intervention; they should allow for comparisons between different service deliveries; they should reflect appropriately the changes in the domains that are being targeted by the treatment; they should assist communication between professions, patients and relatives, and health purchasers.

INVESTIGATING WHETHER THE WHO CLASSIFICATION WOULD HELP TO IDENTIFY THERAPY GOALS

A study of outcome measurement must essentially start by having a full understanding the goals of a particular service. This can then act as the benchmark to see whether the stated goals have been achieved (Langton Hewer, 1990). According to many authorities, physiotherapy, occupational therapy, rehabilitation nursing aim to:

- *improve/remediate the underlying impairment;* for example, treat impaired muscle tone, improve range of movement, increase balance, and alleviate a pressure area;
- *extend functional performance;* for example, by encouraging adapted methods in the activities of daily living or by increasing independence by introducing and encouraging the appropriate use of environmental aids and appliances;
- *improve social integration;* for example, by developing strategies to limit the personal and social disadvantage of the deficit by clients and caregivers;
- *alleviate emotional distress;* for example, by supporting the client and caregivers during the adjustment phase.

To establish whether the World Health Association (WHO) classification would be appropriate for consideration for development as a model for outcomes, the case notes from 300 persons attending therapy were examined. The goals within these notes were identified and a large majority could be included under the groupings of impairment, disability, and handicap. **There were no client groups that did not have goals attributed to all of these sections.** There was one group of goals identified by therapists that were difficult to mesh with this classification; these related to the emotional well-being of clients and their families. Therapists frequently try to reduce anxiety, depression, anger, and fear and improve control and emotional coping strategies. As so many goals were identified in this area, it was felt important to extend the classification by adding the heading of **"distress/well-being"** for the purposes of this study. The importance of addressing emotional state in health care delivery was identified two decades ago by Rosser (1976), who suggested this as an outcome measurement. Subsequent studies have found that well-being is an important factor in noting significant clinical change (Gamiats, Palinkas, & Kaplan, 1992; Long, 1996; Paterson 1996).

Despite this broad range of goals, the majority of therapists were using assessments that targeted pathological dysfunction alone, rendering it difficult to monitor the other treatment objectives. One of the essential components with regard to this approach is the acknowledgment that therapy endeavors to impact on many areas of the client's life and thus the outcome measure must reflect this broad range of domains.

Wood and Badley (1978) and Wood (1980) identified that health care systems across the world were frequently attempting to have a broader impact than purely the reduction and prevention of disease. They developed a language, adopted by the World Health Organization, which could reflect an extension to the sequence of events underlying illness-related phenomena. They presented this profile as:

Disease → impairment → disability → handicap.

As therapists are not primarily involved in effecting the pathology/disease, this study has particularly dwelled on capturing aspects related to the impairment, disability, and handicap which are defined in Table 1–1.

Table 1-1. World Health Organization's definitions of impairment, disability and handicap.

IMPAIRMENT	Dysfunction resulting from pathological changes in system
DISABILITY	Consequence of impairment in terms of functional performance (disturbance at level of person)
HANDICAP	Disadvantages experienced by the individual as a result of impairment and disabilities; reflects interaction with and adaptation to the individual's surroundings

This form of classification[1] allows one to reflect on the different impacts on the health of an individual. For example, some conditions will "impair" slightly but cause severe "disability" and "handicap." whereas others may show major "impairment" but limited "disability" and "handicap," Therapists are frequently struck by those whose lives have been severely affected by what may appear to be a mild impairment whereas others may overcome major disorders so that they live independent and rewarding lives.

Since Wood and Badley's work in 1978, there has been considerable discussion with regard to the aspect of emotional distress/well-being associated with disease and dysfunction. It is possible that the revision of the international classification of Impairment, Disability, and Handicap will extend and include this domain. We found in the study of therapy goals that frequently there were goals associated with improving the emotional status of the patient and relatives and therefore this domain has to be identified separately. After all, if a rehabilitation program for a severely disabled person is focused on improving his or her adjustment and coping strategies, it is important to be able to identify whether this is achieved. Many treatises on the effectiveness of health service provision, rehabilitation, and outcome dwell on the importance

[1]A revision of the International Classification of Impairment, Disability, and Handicap officially commenced in 1993 and was coordinated by the WCC WHO Collaborating Centre, Nationale Road voor de Volksgezondheid, P.O. Box 7100, 2701 AC Zoetmeer, Netherlands.

of "quality of life" (Rosser 1976). Although this term has become increasingly fashionable, it has not been defined (McKenna, Hunt, & Tennant, 1993). Therapists feel strongly that they contribute to improving this elusive *je ne sais quoi*, but in this study we have avoided the use of the term "quality of life" as it lacks specificity and can be interpreted in too many ways. However, the essentials of this concept are probably captured in the domains of handicap and distress/well-being. Interestingly, no goals specifying "improving quality of life" were found in the case notes study but goals associated with "improving self esteem," "improving personal autonomy," "teaching coping strategies to reduce fear" and "helping a person to come to terms" were mentioned frequently.

A revision of the International Classification of Impairment, Disability, and Handicap (ICIDH) officially commenced in 1993 and is being coordinated by the WCC WHO Collaborating Centre in the Netherlands. This revision started after the beginning of our work in using the ICIDH for this project. However, from the materials that are presently available, it appears that the new revision will not affect the approach that we have taken. The Dutch Collaborating Centre has announced that the three main concepts of the ICIDH will now be termed "Dimensions" and has clarified the definitions related to these. Thus the definition of "impairment" is being suggested to be "a loss or abnormality of body structure or of physiological or psychological function." The definition of the dimension of "disability" will be redefined as one of "activity" which is clarified as "something a person does, ranging from very basic, elementary, or simple to complex. Difficulties in performing activities occur when there is a qualitative or quantitative alteration in the way which these activities are carried out." The domain of "handicap" is suggested to be renamed as either "participation" or "social participation" and is defined as "the nature and extent of a person's involvement in life situations in relationship to impairments, activities, and contextual factors." The Beta version of ICIDH was piloted during 1997 and it is hoped that the revised ICIDH-2 will be presented to the World Health Assembly in 1999 (Ustun, B. News on the ICIDH. Centre for Standard of Informatics in Health Care; *Newsletter, 4*, 2–7).

Despite high level, far reaching, lengthy, and international debate there will probably never be a totally acceptable model of disability. The medical model and the social model have their places and offer components that facilitate the understanding of the needs of disabled people at different times. Therapists do not necessarily feel entirely comfortable with either as they are aware that "illness," "disease," and "dysfunction" are psychophysiological processes that limit the person's coping abilities (Fugl-Meyer, Brandholm, & Fugl-Meyer, 1991). This philosophy is core to one of the aims of rehabilitation, which is to mobilize the resources of an individual so that, by having realistic goals and adapting physically and psychologically, they may achieve optimal life satisfaction. This approach is supported by McCrae and Costa (1986), who found that patients who used effective coping strategies reported higher subsequent life satisfaction. These authors, along with many others (e.g., Frattali, 1991; Stephen & Hetu, 1992; Whiteneck et al. 1992) support the classification of impairment, disability, and handicap as one that can reflect the complexity of the challenges in rehabilitation, but we suggest the addition of adding the concept of distress/well-being in its own right rather than being embedded within the other domains.

Studies have indicated poor correlations between the impairments, disabilities, and handicaps in some individuals from particular client groups. For example, in heart failure there may be no relation between cardiac output (impairment) with treadmill exercise tolerance, timed walking tests (disabilities/activities), and social activity (handicap/participation) (Cowley et al., 1991). This lack of direct relationship between impairment, disability, and handicap also applies in chronic airway disease (Williams & Bury, 1989).

From the patients' point of view, impairment may be of less importance than the restrictions these place on everyday life. The following four case histories illustrate the different impact of different disorders.

CASE STUDY 1: MR.SP

IMPAIRMENT	Mr. SP has had a stroke, he has a mild hemiplegia with some loss of dexterity in his left hand and increased tone in his left leg.
DISABILITY/ACTIVITY	Mr. SP is able to undertake all tasks for himself but prefers his wife to help him with most activities. He requires extra time and encouragement in all daily living activities.
HANDICAP/PARTICIPATION	Mr. SP has become extremely passive, his dominant wife has taken over all household and social tasks. He has retired early and withdrawn from previously enjoyed social activities.
DISTRESS/WELL-BEING	Mr. SP has become depressed and anxious, fearing another stroke, feeling old and as if life has nothing to offer him. His wife is extremely irritated and anxious, concerned that he may deteriorate if he exerts himself and worried about what the future may hold.
SUMMARY	Mr. SP has what may be considered a mild impairment with moderate disability and severe social (handicap) and emotional consequence.

CASE STUDY 2: MRS. PR

IMPAIRMENT	Mrs. PR has had multiple sclerosis for 15 years. She is severely ataxic and has increased tone in all limbs. Her sitting balance is poor.
DISABILITY/ACTIVITY	Mrs. PR uses an adapted wheelchair and all aids and appliances in the home effectively. She is in an adapted accommodation and can get to the local shops. She is able to care for the house, provide meals for the family, and communicate effectively.
HANDICAP/PARTICIPATION	Mrs. PR plays an active social role, she is a school governor as well as acting on the local community health council. She enjoys her garden and wheelchair dancing.
DISTRESS/WELL-BEING	Mrs. PR is a determined, resourceful lady who, not surprisingly, becomes concerned and frustrated on some occasions but is generally positive and uses good emotional support strategies.
SUMMARY	Mrs. PR has a severe level of impairment but overcomes most functional restrictions using resourcefulness and appropriate aids; thus, she is only partially disabled. She is not socially handicapped in any specific way.

CASE STUDY 3: MR. K

IMPAIRMENT	Mr. K has a mild expressive and receptive language disorder (dysphasia/aphasia).
DISABILITY/ACTIVITY	Although speaking quite freely, he has difficulty in making himself understood quickly in a group of people or over the telephone. Mr. K occasionally misunderstands meanings, particularly if there is a rapid change of subject. He is dependent on others being attentive and patient listeners.
HANDICAP/PARTICIPATION	Mr. K is now unable to be employed, as he had been previously; he has withdrawn from social settings and has given up all hobbies and no longer contributes to decision making.
SUMMARY	This gentleman could be seen as having a mild impairment, a moderate disability, and quite a severe social handicap.[2]

[2]Handicap/Participation according to the ICD classification is not classified according to individuals or their attributes but rather according to the circumstances in which disabled people are likely to find themselves, circumstances that can be expected to place such individuals at a disadvantage in relation to their peers when viewed from the norms of society. The scheme is not exhaustive and is restricted to key social roles that have been regarded as the most important dimensions of disadvantages—social integration, occupation, economic self-sufficiency.

CASE STUDY 4: MR. C

IMPAIRMENT	Mr. C, a 40-year-old gentleman who has cerebral palsy and is wheelchair bound. Mr. C is quadriplegic and dysarthric.
DISABILITY/ACTIVITY	Mr. C is totally independent, using an adapted wheelchair and living in adapted accommodation. He can communicate in all situations with a communication aid with special adaptations for the telephone.
HANDICAP/PARTICIPATION	Mr. C is employed as a solicitor and is an active member in the disability movement; he has a full work and social life and his views are sought and valued by a number of contacts.
SUMMARY	This gentleman, who has a very severe level of impairment, has been able to overcome his difficulties so that functionally, although restricted, he is independent and he is not socially handicapped in any particular way.

CHAPTER 2

Methodology

The authors initially developed the Therapy Outcome Measures (TOM) for speech and language therapists (see Enderby 1992; Enderby & John, 1997). Subsequently work was undertaken to develop and trial this approach for use by physiotherapists, occupational therapists, and rehabilitation nurses. Further trials to establish its appropriateness for podiatrists is underway.

A primary core scale was developed. The points on the scale reflect specific concepts related to the levels within each domain of impairment, disability, handicap, distress/well-being. These identified principles that should be fundamental and should be reflected in the clients' specific scales (See Appendix 1). Ten hospitals and community trusts of physiotherapists and occupational therapists participated in the study. Each group was asked to develop definitions that would reflect the abilities/difficulties found by patients in different client groups at different levels on the core scale. Thus, therapists were asked to describe patients who had mild, moderate, or severe impairments, disabilities, and handicaps. The client groups chosen for the study reflected the expertise and interests of the therapists involved. The scales generated by the different working groups were then circulated so that therapists deleted terms or chose others, achieving a consensus with regard to the terminology at each point on all the scales. This Modified Delphi technique of eliciting and feeding back information led to definitions acceptable to therapists working in different facilities with a broad range of clients.

The definitions in the specific scales aim to achieve a method of communicating views of therapists about the severity and nature of the presentation within a domain, thus in essence they attempt to clarify what is meant by "severe," "moderate," "mild," and so forth. The descriptors should prompt the therapist to help with the best match, that is, my "patient is most like that." It is unlikely that any patient will fit precisely within any descriptor or have all the deficits or abilities represented in the scale description. Therapists generally unconsciously rank patients, for example, "he is a bit better than her," "she is the worst I have seen with this disorder," and so forth. The scale score attempts to make the judgments more explicit.

The detailed scales (Appendix 2) reflected the core scale principles in an amplified way in order to reflect the terminology commonly used by practicing clinicians to describe the performance and abilities at the different levels. Within any profession there are different schools of thought and whenever possible these have been accommodated; for example, there are different views with regard to the underlying cause of dyspraxia and its resultant representations. The philosophy underpinning this project is that the scales should not "lead" any therapists but allow clinical judgment to be reflected. Thus the concepts of core scales are important and the detailed scales are used to facilitate achieving reliability in clinical judgments by being more precise in defining levels of severity or ability

RELIABILITY

The four domain scales are on an 11-point ordinal scale with zero representing the most severe category and 5, normal. Each integer (0–5) has a corresponding description and a score of .5 indicates that the subject is slightly better or worse than the description. To assess the interobserver reliability of these scales the expected agreement by chance needs to be considered, and a method is needed that takes into consideration that a disagreement from say 1 to 1.5 is not as serious as a disagreement from 1 to 2. A suitable chance corrected measure of reliability when there are two observers that takes into consideration the seriousness of different disagreements is the weighted Kappa (Cohen, 1968). The question then arises over what are suitable weights for the weighted Kappa "unless there are strong prior reasons, the most commonly used weighting scheme, called quadratic weights, which bases disagreement weights on the square of the amount of discrepancy, should be used" (Streiner & Norman, 1989).

By using quadratic weights the weighted Kappa is identical to the intraclass correlation coefficient (Streiner & Norman, 1989). Maclure and Willett (1987) concluded that "weighted Kappa is best when it equals the intra-class correlation coefficient." Therefore, the 11 categories in the ordinal scale have been assigned discrete values of 1 (more severe) to 11 (normal), quadratic weights in effect quantify these values.

There are two main questions of interest. First, what is the overall group reliability of the therapists on each scale and second, for training purposes, what is the reliability of each individual observer with respect to the other observers in that group? There is no observer in the groups who could be taken as a standard, thus to answer the second question it is necessary to look at the interobserver reliability between each pair of observers within the group.

Groups of therapists—19 speech therapists, 15 occupational therapists, and 14 physiotherapists—were introduced to the therapy outcome measure in 1½ hour training sessions. Each profession had separate training sessions that used examples related particularly to their areas of interest. The training familiarized the therapists with the concepts related to impairment, disability, handicap, and well-being and provided time for individual therapists to practice scoring. The reliability trial required the therapists to score patients, without collusion, having been presented case histories (written and verbal) supported by audio- and video-tape. Each therapist was allowed to ask the presenter for clarification of any particular fact.

The patients were chosen to represent a broad range of difficulty, thus persons with different types and degree of impairments and disabilities were chosen. For the pairwise interobserver reliability, in essence a two observer problem, quadratic weights were assigned so that the weighted Kappa equals the intraclass correlation coefficient. The coefficient that was used is taken from Streiner and Norman (1989) and is defined by:

$$R = \frac{\sigma^2 \text{ subject}}{\sigma^2 \text{ subject} + \sigma^2 \text{ observers} + \sigma^2 \text{ error}}$$

Therapists who did not rate all the subjects were removed from the analysis.

Landis and Koch (1977) recommended the following interpretations for reliability coefficients (Table 2–1):

Table 2–1. Benchmarks for the interpretation of observed Kappa values.

Kappa Statistic	Strength of Agreement
<0.00	Poor
0.00–0.20	Slight
0.21–0.40	Fair
0.41–0.60	Moderate
0.61–0.80	Substantial
0.81–1.00	Almost Perfect

RESULTS

Occupational Therapists

Fifteen occupational therapists participated and scored subjects. Five occupational therapists had incomplete ratings. Thus, 10 occupational therapists' results were used for the analysis. In addition, one further occupational therapist missed ratings for Subjects 3 and 4 for the well-being scale only. Therefore, this occupational therapist's results were removed from the reliability analysis for the well-being scale only.

Table 2–2. Interobserver reliability of the occupational therapists.

	Impairment	Disability	Handicap	Well-being
ICC	0.84	0.85	0.74	0.58

Physiotherapists

Fourteen physiotherapists scored five subjects. Two physiotherapists gave incomplete data and thus the results of 12 physiotherapists are reported.

Table 2–3. Interobserver reliability of the physiotherapists.

	Impairment	Disability	Handicap	Well-being
ICC	0.66	0.74	0.77	0.57

Speech Therapists

Nineteen speech therapists judged six subjects. Three gave incomplete data and were excluded from analysis. A further four therapists did not rate well-being on all clients and were removed from the reliability analysis of the well-being scale.

Table 2–4. Interobserver reliability of the speech therapists.

	Impairment	Disability	Handicap	Well-being
ICC	0.89	0.90	0.84	0.57

There are several points to note with regard to the reliability trial. We had considerable difficulty in establishing an appropriate method of reflecting the well-being of the patient and carer. Case histories and audio recordings do not necessarily capture the mood of the patient and thus therapists were left to surmise with very little information. It would appear from subsequent trials that the therapists involved have found it much easier to score well-being when they personally know a patient and have more detailed information on which to make a judgment.

The physiotherapists had some difficulty in judging the impairment of patients by observation alone. Issues to do with tone, movement to resistance, and reflexes were not reflected in the material. We would suggest that the slightly reduced interobserver reliability of the physiotherapists in this trial underestimates the potential reliability in a normal clinical situation.

A further eight therapists were recruited to examine reliability when presented with amplified clinical information. More detailed information was given to the eight therapists who were allowed to examine and question the patient and carer in each others' presence but were instructed not to collude over ratings. The results of this trial are presented in Table 2–5.

Table 2–5. The overall group reliability of the therapists on the four scales.

	Impairment	Disability	Handicap	Well-being of	
				Client	Carer
ICC	0.87	0.77	0.66	0.73	0.75

Pairwise comparisons of the therapists are presented in Tables 2–6, 2–7, 2–8, 2–9, and 2–10.

Table 2–6 Pairwise intertherapist agreement for the impairment scale.

	T1	T2	T3	T4	T5	T6	T7	T8
T1	—	0.96	0.87	0.84	0.91	0.96	0.94	0.97
T2		—	0.85	0.80	0.94	0.95	0.93	0.92
T3			—	0.78	0.81	0.86	0.80	0.96
T4				—	0.58	0.86	0.71	0.83
T5					—	0.89	0.93	0.88
T6						—	0.89	0.93
T7							—	0.89
T8	(Symmetric)							—

Table 2–7. Pairwise intertherapist agreement for the disability scale.

	T1	T2	T3	T4	T5	T6	T7	T8
T1	—	0.73	0.73	0.77	0.83	0.76	0.91	0.62
T2		—	0.75	0.72	0.82	0.61	0.71	0.85
T3			—	0.91	0.90	0.71	0.65	0.83
T4				—	0.87	0.93	0.68	0.84
T5					—	0.71	0.72	0.90
T6						—	0.67	0.70
T7							—	0.53
T8	(Symmetric)							—

Table 2–8 Pairwise intertherapist agreement for the handicap scale.

	T1	T2	T3	T4	T5	T6	T7	T8
T1	—	0.54	0.25	0.50	0.38	0.30	0.54	0.35
T2		—	0.71	0.94	0.93	0.27	1.00	0.79
T3			—	0.72	0.81	0.24	0.71	0.83
T4				—	0.94	0.24	0.94	0.92
T5					—	0.24	0.93	0.87
T6						—	0.27	0.19
T7							—	0.79
T8	(Symmetric)							—

Note: Therapist 1 has fair to moderate agreement with the other therapists. Therapist 6 has fair agreement.

Table 2–9. Pairwise intertherapist agreement on the well-being of the client.

	T1	T2	T3	T4	T5	T6	T7	T8
T1	—	0.56	0.64	0.48	0.73	0.43	0.82	0.73
T2		—	0.51	0.83	0.86	0.67	0.79	0.64
T3			—	0.72	0.78	0.63	0.78	0.90
T4				—	0.89	0.79	0.85	0.82
T5					—	0.69	0.96	0.84
T6						—	0.67	0.68
T7							—	0.82
T8	(Symmetric)							—

Table 2–10. Pairwise intertherapist agreement on the well-being of the carer.

	T1	T2	T3	T4	T5	T6	T7	T8
T1	—	0.71	0.49	0.62	0.76	0.67	0.96	0.49
T2		—	0.66	0.65	0.91	0.88	0.85	0.63
T3			—	0.85	0.69	0.84	0.63	0.98
T4				—	0.82	0.82	0.72	0.88
T5					—	0.89	0.88	0.70
T6						—	0.85	0.86
T7							—	0.64
T8	(Symmetric)							—

Undertaking clinical reliability studies with patients is difficult. There are concerns about exposing patients and their relatives to a group of observers who independently assess and gauge the responses on a range of tasks. However, video and audio information, along with case notes, can be either inadequate or reveal information in such a way as to prime the judges. Many reliability studies have been comprised of the relationship between the scores of two independent judges assessing an individual patient; however, this does not give sufficient information to look at the range of agreement/disagreement in a broad range of observers who have different skills, backgrounds, and philosophies. In developing this tool different methods of interrater reliability trial have been conducted over the years. In essence, these studies would suggest a high degree of reliability in the areas of impairment and disability and good reliability in the areas of handicap and well-being.

VALIDITY

A measure is only valid to the extent that it measures what it purports to measure (Wilkin, Hallam, & Doggett, 1992). In validating a measure, there is a need to determine the degree of confidence that can be placed on the inferences drawn from the individual's scores on that measure. In other words, can one believe what the measure indicates?

The literature describes three classic ways of ascertaining validity, namely, content, criterion, and construct. Validity can be measured by ascertaining the degree to which what has been measured corresponds with other independent measures obtained by different research tools. At present there are not really any comparable measures to the TOM that could be used as a "gold" standard. Therefore it is not possible to use criterion validity, with its requirement that the results of the measure be compared with another. Nor can construct validity be used because there is not, as yet, sufficient knowledge of the pattern of relationships, regarding the distribution of scores among different groups, to allow comparisons. Therefore, face and content validity are the descriptions of validity that have been addressed.

FACE VALIDITY

Face validity concerns whether, on the face of it, the measure captures the qualities to be measured. The criterion for assessing face validity rests on the subjective judgment that is based on a review of the measure; that the selection of items appears sensible, in the view of a panel of experts. Guilford (1954) described this approach to validation as "validation by assumption"; that the instrument measures "such and such" because an expert says it does.

Content validity concerns whether the domain of content is relevant to the measure, whether the items included in the domain are a representative sample of the target behaviors. Appropriate content is more likely if a number of representative judges are used to generate and select the items for the scales, and, if the content included is regarded as important, as supported through the literature. Demonstration of content validity rests mainly on an "appeal to reason" in respect to the adequacy with which the domain has been defined.

Acceptance of the face and content validity of the TOM was based on a review by an "expert" panel, comprised of therapists working within the particular specialties covered by the measure.

The TOM comprises a core scale. In order to facilitate decision making and reliability of judgment, adaptations were made to the core scales. These adaptations provided operational descriptions for whole points on the scale. Therapists specializing in different client groups from different health districts contributed to the content of the scales through use of the Delphi technique. The differing scales that were developed were then amalgamated to form an agreed-on "set."

The TOM, as adapted for occupational therapy and physiotherapy patient groups, was used in the study to assess the validity of the information gained over a period of time. It aimed to assess whether the TOM provides valid and reliable information on the changes effected during intervention. This was done by feeding back the data to the therapists and ascertaining whether the results obtained did reflect typical changes effected in their patients, and whether the results could be used to inform therapists and to allow them to make inferences from the data. Face validity was established from this method.

CHAPTER 3

Operational Instructions

The reliability of this approach is dependent on:

- Having a clear understanding of the concepts of impairment, disability, handicap, and distress. It may assist you to discuss these concepts with colleagues to improve familiarity;
- Reading the operational manual and becoming comfortable with the core scale and the details of specific scales;
- Practicing on at least 10 patients prior to collecting any data that you can rely on. Remember that at first it may take you 10 to 15 minutes to score a patient but after a little practice most therapists report that the procedure takes less than 3 minutes and they become more confident in making judgments;
- Having a group rating session where clinical decisions on rating can be compared and discussed to improve understanding of the issues. Practical and logistic aspects of implementing the approach, e.g., who is going to collect and aggregate the data, what time points are appropriate, should be agreed at the outset.

WHAT WILL I GET OUT OF THIS? DATA ANALYSIS

Prior to making the decision to use this or any other outcome measure, it is important to consider whether the data that is to be generated will be accessible and informative.

Obviously it is hoped that each therapist will be informed about the progress of each client that he or she is seeing if he or she collects and peruses the individual results. However, the data will be more informative if it is collected in a way enabling aggregation and analysis in the context of variables that may influence outcome, for example, age and diagnosis.

It is vital to consider the method of data collection and analysis at an early opportunity. Preferably this should be done with local agreement with the appropriate managers and the arrangements should be clear before the technique is adopted.

The research underpinning this project led to the development of software that can run on a PC and generates data compatible with Access. The software restricts the user to the codes and fields of information given in the appendices.

If, locally, you wish to incorporate outcome data with an existing information system, then the codes and other existing related fields may need adaptation, but you will need to discuss adding fields to allow the outcome scores to be input and the report specification that will be changed by adding outcome as a parameter. Consider how you will collect information, how it will be entered, and how you will get information out.

WHICH PATIENTS SHOULD I USE THIS ON?

Most research investigating the impact of therapy has included relatively small specific cohorts of patients. The necessity of tight selection criteria in research has led to difficulties regarding the representativeness of the results. For example, most research studies relating to therapy for stroke patients have included younger patients who have had no previous stroke or neurological pathology, whereas therapists commonly treat older patients with complex past medical histories. Gathering outcome data on all patients completing an episode of therapy should furnish us all with more representative data to examine treatment outcomes.

Outcome data should be collected on all patients who are receiving therapy. The results are often more informative when there are larger groups of patients and the data can be aggregated and an individual's performance can be compared with that of the group. Outcome data cannot be collected on patients who attend therapy for advice alone unless there is a follow-up appointment, or audit survey, to see whether the advice has influenced any of the domains. In essence it is important for the patient to attend the initial appointment/s in order that the patient's status can be reflected in the first score and, at an appointment at a later stage, for one to be able to gauge any change. Thus if a patient does not appear for follow-up appointments then it is impossible to collect this information!

HOW OFTEN SHOULD I SCORE A PATIENT?

The minimum requirements for outcome measurement are to evaluate performance at the beginning and end of an episode of care. An episode of care may be determined when the patient is to be discharged, put on review, transferred from intensive to individual therapy, starting a program using particular aids or equipment, or the goals of therapy are changing. However, there are many client groups receiving therapy who have long periods of intervention and it is recommended that these patients are monitored on a 6-month basis. Some purchaser contracts may specify different requirements. The first score on a patient is called the Admissions score (A), the end/beginning of a new episode of care is called the Intermediate score (I) and when the patient is discharged from further therapy the score is entitled Final (F).

HOW DO I CHOOSE A POINT ON THE SCALE?

The descriptions on the scales are unlikely to fit any particular client specifically. They provide descriptions of a range of behaviors that are present at that point on the scale. Therefore choose the elements of relevance to the patient. It is important to match the client to the description that is the "best fit," despite the fact that the client may not have all the parameters stated or may have others that are unstated. The descriptors are meant to give the general impression of the level of difficulty. They are to assist a therapist to reflect her/his clinical opinion with regard to the patient's status.

If new information becomes available and suggests that the wrong scale point was chosen, then this may be amended retrospectively. For example, on first attendance, emotions may be concealed and a patient may only admit to severe frustration/depression once he has become more comfortable with the therapist. Thus a retrospective scaling down of that particular domain is appropriate to reflect the clinical opinion that has altered, given this new information.

If you are seeing patients from client groups that are not covered by the scales presented here then you may use the core scale in Appendix 1 or you may wish to use the most appropriate similar scale, that is the best fit, or adapt a scale or develop one of your own. If you adapt or develop a scale the authors will be happy to inspect it and consider authorizing its use.

Using Half Points

If a client is better or worse than the descriptor then the half point (.5) is used to reflect the direction that is appropriate. For example, if the client is a little better than the descriptor on the scale point 3, but not as good as scale point 4, then select 3.5.

COMPLETING THE DATA ENTRY FORM

The data entry form that was used in the research is shown in Appendix 4. These forms can be freely photocopied or the specific domains can be integrated in an existing local data information system. Brief notes to prompt the correct completion on the forms is given in Appendix 6. According to the analyses that you wish to undertake, the information you need to collect should be considered. For example, if you wish to examine outcome measures by individual therapists then it will be necessary to enter the therapist's name on the top of the form and to have an appropriate field in your database to reflect this. If you do not wish to do this, but want to look at outcome measures by profession, then you need only identify "physiotherapist," "occupational therapist," or "rehabilitation nurse."

If you wish to analyze outcome data by date of birth, then it will be necessary for you to detail on the form the age of the patient in years under the patient's details. If you wish to analyze the information of outcomes related to duration of treatment, then you will need to fill in the amount of treatment that the patient achieved when the final score is detailed. It is essential that the details of these requirements are agreed on with the other therapists in your locality who are participating in the collection of outcomes. You should all be completing the data form in an agreed-on manner to ensure you all comply consistently.

Most outcome measure results will need grouping according to the medical diagnosis and the therapy/nursing diagnosis. The medical diagnosis in this project was termed the **etiology** and the etiology codes used in this research project are listed in Appendix 3. The physiotherapy, occupational therapy, and rehabilitation nursing diagnoses are termed **disorder** and are listed in the same appendix. If you are analyzing data locally then you may wish to amend the etiologies or impairment codes and program your computer accordingly.

You will note that there is a space for two disorder codes on the data collection form. Identify the most relevant in the first space. The first score that you undertake on patients should be identified by an (A) when you first **assess** them or they are **admitted** to treatment. The initial assessment to an episode of care may only be arrived at after a few appointments but should be entered prior to the treatment beginning. To comply with the philosophy of this approach, which is to reflect the therapist's clinical judgment, it is allowable to amend this "assessment" score if subsequent information is elicited that would amend the clinical view, for example, if a patient initially denies any functional deficit but later details such difficulties. In this event the therapist may wish to amend the "A" score for disability, downward. Place the relevant scores in the box for impairment, disability, handicap, and well-being/distress. If there is a change in episode of care then an "I" score denotes the intermediate score when the patient is being reviewed. There may be several intermediate "I" scores. The final score should be identified by "F." If the patient, at any stage, has an intervening illness or event and needs a new course of therapy, then enter the "I" score reflecting the status prior to the event and then start a new "A" score which can be used to identify the change.

RATING

Select a rating to most closely reflect the level of ability the client has. Do not forget to use the half point (.5) to indicate if a patient is slightly better/worse than the descriptor. Score two "impairment" scores if this is appropriate. The first impairment score should relate to the most relevant difficulty in this episode of care. Where there are more than two impairments choose "multifactorial" scale and code.

WELL-BEING/DISTRESS

Health care staff frequently offer support and encouragement, trying to influence the well-being/distress of the patient along with their families or carers. In order to capture information in this domain a specific scale has been developed. During the pilot studies, reported elsewhere, it became evident that it was necessary to rate the well-being of the patient and relatives/carers separately, thus the well-being/distress of the client (first space) and carer (second space) can be separately reflected.

WHAT HAPPENS IF THE PATIENTS/ RELATIVES APPEAR TO GET WORSE?

Therapists frequently feel uncomfortable in reflecting a deterioration in the patient's ability. It is not uncommon in some client groups for patients' impairments to worsen despite therapy involvement. In some circumstances the well-being of patient and carer may worsen during the course of the disorder as realization of the implications of the disorder impinge. Outcome measures cannot change the status quo and it is important to reflect the situation as it is. By gathering information on large groups of patients, it is possible to identify common patterns associated with different disorders. For example, some children may have age-appropriate disability, handicap, and well-being when they are infants but as their peer group develops, the gap between them and their peer group becomes greater, thus giving the appearance of the child becoming more disabled and handicapped. This of course reflects the true situation.

AGREEMENT SCORE/USER INVOLVEMENT

Determining the most appropriate way of ensuring that information captures patients' and relatives' views regarding the outcome of therapy has been challenging. Separate work is being undertaken where patients and relatives are completing outcome scales independently of therapists to study the degree of consensus. At the present time, however, the most appropriate way of proceeding is for the intermediate and/or the final scores to be discussed with the patient and relatives to establish whether the patient and relatives agree with the therapist in their summary of the situation. The agreement scale originally had five points but has more recently been reduced to three (see Table 3–1).

It is not appropriate for a therapist to use the terms "impairment," "disability," "handicap," "distress/well-being" with patients and relatives, but the information can be elicited by talking about the specific physical and/or psychological problem in terms that are familiar to the patient; what it prevents them from doing and what they are able to do; and the consequences on their general lifestyle along with how this affects them emotionally. This can be done in a gentle and open way and the views of the therapist, with regard to gains, can be tested against the views of the patient and the relative.

It is acknowledged that this approach is somewhat crude but it has been found to be of value to therapists who are sometimes unaware of the different perceptions of the patients and/or relatives with regard to the gains made.

Table 3–1. Agreement score.

1. Professional/client/caregiver do not agree on outcome.

2. Professional/client/caregiver do not agree equally on outcome.

3. Professional/client/caregiver agree on outcome in all domains.

Note: Agreement relates to agreed view even when there is no change in any domain, that is, client, caregiver, or professional may have total agreement that nothing has changed.

CAVEATS

It is not difficult to criticize this approach to outcome measurement. Trying to capture and reflect clinical judgment in an organized and systematic way is bound to cause difficulties particularly related to subjectivity, sensitivity, and reliability. However, we feel strongly that this approach holds promise—improving our collection of outcome data in a practical, reliable, achievable, communicable manner and allowing for the pooling of information related to clinical experience and different service delivery patterns.

LOCAL TRAINING IN USING TOM

We strongly advise that, prior to using TOM, groups of staff get together to agree on certain principles in its usage and to ensure that each staff member has a good understanding of the philosophical underpinning and practical issues in application.

The group discussion may be assisted by following this format:

- Discussion regarding need for outcome measurement
- Discussion regarding dimensions of impairment, disability, handicap, and well-being
- Practice in rating patients (see below for suggestions)

■ Practice in completing forms and coding
■ Agreement on:
  · pilot/trial study period
  · who to score (which patient group - all or particular ones)
  · who/how to analyze data
  · who/how to train new staff members
  · when to review information

It is essential for the success of any such outcome initiative to have a clearly defined and agreed action plan that reflects the whole project.

PRACTICE ON CASE STUDIES

Therapists and nurses can practice applying the TOM scoring in different ways. One approach that we would suggest follows:

A therapist/nurse presents a case study. The patient should be well known to them. They should outline

■ age
■ medical etiology
■ the condition, detailing severity and complicating factors
■ what the patient is able/unable to do for him/herself, activities of daily living
■ social circumstances, social disadvantages, participation
■ emotional state

All other participants may ask questions of the presenter until they feel comfortable scoring. The group should score the patient independently using the core scale and learning prompt sheet (see Appendix 7). When everyone has completed scoring they should share the scores with the group. The participants who have attributed scores at variance with the group should explain their reasoning. It is unlikely that all those involved will agree on a precise score. However, one wishes to achieve agreement by 80% of the group within one whole point.

Each member then gives a further presentation in the same way, but this time the persons scoring should use the detailed core scale suggested as being appropriate. This approach to training has been found to provide therapists with a familiarity and understanding of the scale. It develops consensus in judgments using the scale and develops reliability in using the measure.

CHAPTER 4

Clinical Trial Results

This prospective study examined the use of the Therapy Outcome Measure over a 9-month period, in a variety of clinical settings. Six occupational therapy departments and eight physiotherapy departments agreed to participate in the study. All new patients referred to these departments within the study period were included. If the patient was discharged within the 9-month period their final score at point of discharge was taken. For those patients still currently on the books at the end of the 9-month period, a score was taken at that time. Thus the data presented here include some patients who had not completed their course of treatment.

All therapists involved in the study had participated in at least one half-day training, either carried out by the authors or by named trainers. They had been involved in the exercises and practice as detailed in this manual. Results relating to the first 10 patients that they scored were not included in the study analysis so that the results presented were derived from people who have had a degree of experience in using the method. For the purposes of this manual we have selected the results related to client groups with significant numbers of patients. Further data related to this study will be submitted for publication elsewhere.

OCCUPATIONAL THERAPY

A total of 550 patients, representing a broad range of etiologies and impairments, were included in the study. A total of 31 occupational therapists submitted forms. Of these 550 patients, 137 had more than one impairment and 124 cases had carer well-being noted.

Combined Scores for All Client Groups—Occupational Therapy

The average number of contacts for the 550 patients was 13.4 and these were spread over an average duration of 3.15 months. The average start, change, and finish scores for each domain are represented in Table 4–1.

Table 4–1. Average Start, Change, and Finish Scores for each domain: Occupational Therapy ($N = 550$).

	F1	D	H	PWB	CWB ($N = 124$)
Start	2.63	2.65	2.6	2.85	3.45
Change	0.45	0.45	0.45	0.5	0.5
Finish	3.1	3.15	3.05	3.4	4

In such a heterogeneous group of patients one would expect that some patients will deteriorate in some domains whereas others may make great gains. Table 4–2 illustrates that in each domain between 6% and 8% of patients deteriorated and a further 43% of patients showed no change. However, between a third and just under half of patients changed between .5 and 1 point on the scale. (see Table 4–2). Clinicians would expect that some patients would change in all five domains whereas others may change in just one or two domains, showing a more specific effect. Table 4–3 demonstrates that, of the 550 patients, only 42 did not change in any domain but more than half (53.5%) of patients changed in three or more domains. (see Table 4–3).

Table 4–2. Percentage of patients with change amount: Occupational Therapy ($N = 550$).

	F1	D	H	PWB	CWB ($N = 124$)
Negative	7.5	5.9	6.4	6.8	6.4
None	43.7	41	41.6	41.6	42.7
0.5–1	38	41.8	43.2	39.2	38.7
1.5–2	9	10	7.5	8.8	7.2
2.5–3	1.6	0.9	1	3	1.6
3.5–5	0	0.1	0	0.3	3.2

Table 4–3. Number of domain changes: Occupational Therapy ($N = 550$).

None	1	2	3	4	5
42	107	109	134	113	42

Client-Specific Groups' Results—Occupational Therapy

Table 4–4 gives the average start, change, and finish scores along with the percentage change for certain etiological groups. For illustrative purposes we have included in Table 4–4 the etiological groups of learning difficulty, mental illness, orthopedic, respiratory disease, acquired neurological—stroke, and frail elderly with multifactorial problems. Percentage change is dependent on the initial score, for example, a small change from a low score is a higher percentage improvement than a small change from a higher base score. The percentage change for this study has been calculated by subtracting the start score from the finish score and dividing by the start score and then multiplying by 100, thus:

Finish − Start ÷ Start × 100 = percentage change

Table 4–4. Occupational Therapy—Average start, change, and finish scores with percentage change for different etiological groups.

Disorder	Number of Subjects	Number with Carer Well-being Score	First Impairment			Disability/ Activity			Handicap/ Participation			Patient Well-being			Carer Well-being		
			S	C %	F	S	C %	F	S	C %	F	S	C %	F	S	C %	F
Learning Difficulties	70	13	2.7	0.05 3.7%	2.8	2.15	0.15 9.3%	2.35	2	0.3 17.5%	2.35	2.4	0.3 12.5%	20.7	3	0.4 13.3%	3.4
Mental Illness	149	6	2.35	0.65 29.8%	3.05	2.5	0.6 26%	3.15	2.3	0.6 26%	2.9	2.1	0.9 42.8%	3	3.65	0.4 10.9%	4.05
Orthopedic	93	22	2.6	0.75 28.8%	3.34	3.15	0.6 19.0%	3.75	3.2	0.5 17.2%	3.75	3.85	0.45 13.0%	4.35	3.95	0.85 21.5%	4.8
Respiratory Disease	76	31	2.45	0.1 4.08%	2.55	2.4	0.3 14.5%	2.75	2.45	0.3 14.5%	2.75	2.85	0.2 7%	3.05	3.34	0.45 13.4%	3.8
Acquired Neurological Stroke	45	22	2.75	0.2 9.0%	3	2.3	0.5 23.9%	2.85	2.3	0.35 23.9%	2.7	2.9	0.25 10.8%	3.2	3.4	0.45 13.2%	3.85
Frail Elderly (multifactorial)	24	8	2.8	0.75 26.7%	3.55	2.75	0.6 21.8%	3.35	2.75	0.45 16.3%	3.2	3.2	0.55 17.2%	3.75	3.6	0.5 13.8%	4.1

Note: S = Start, C = Change, F = Finish

One would probably expect that of those groups the smallest changes in the short period of time (9 months) would be found in the areas of impairment related to learning difficulties and chronic respiratory disease. The results demonstrate that this is the case. Larger changes in the area of impairment are found in mental illness—a change of 29.8%; orthopedic—an impairment change score of 28.8%; and with the frail elderly—an impairment change score of 26.7%.

Disability/activity scores improved quite markedly in all the client groups, apart from learning difficulty, which again showed a low change (9.3%). Again, it would be unlikely with this particular group to show marked change in disability scores over such a short trial period. The disability/activity scores for acquired neurological-stroke showed a gain of 23.9% change despite a low level of change in impairment (9%).

The etiological groups of mental illness and stroke show good gains in the area of handicap/participation with changes of 26% and 23.9%, respectively. The learning difficulties clients do show a more promising change in this domain of 17.5%. This was heartening as many of the clients included in this group were involved in normalization programs that particularly emphasized issues related to this domain, such as participation, being involved in choice, autonomy, role development, and so forth.

Patient well-being was particularly compromised initially in those with mental illness, but over the period of time showed a remarkable change of 42.8%. Patient well-being of those with respiratory disease showed little change (7%) and this is in line with other studies of respiratory disease which have drawn attention to the resistant aspect of patient well-being.

There were surprisingly few patients with carer well-being scores. With some groups this is because a carer was not identifiable or not available to participate in treatment, but with other client groups it is suspected that the therapist did not feel that it was appropriate or necessary to collect information related to this domain. The largest gains related to change in carer well-being were associated with the orthopedic group (21.5%), whereas the gains for those with mental illness (10.9%) were low. However, one must recognize that only six carer well-being scores were collected for this latter group. Do we talk about involving carers in programs of care more than we do it?

Occupational Therapy—Amount of Change

It is likely that a percentage of patients receiving any treatment are either going to show no change or negative change. Also some subjects may well change in one or two domains whereas others may show improvements in all aspects. Table 4–5 identifies the percentage of subjects who have not changed or have negatively changed in any domain, as well as those who have changed in up to two domains. The percentage of patients who have changed in three or more domains is also illustrated.

Small numbers of patients in each group do not change or change in a negative direction. The smallest percentages are found surprisingly in learning difficulties and orthopedic whereas 12% of those with respiratory disease showed negative or no change in any area assessed. More than a third of patients in all the client groups show a positive change in one or two domains and more than 40% of patients in all the groups show broader improvements over time. The most striking group is that of orthopedic, where 61.95% of patients show positive change in three to five domains.

Table 4–5. Occupation Therapy.

Disorder	No. of Subjects	% of Subjects Not Changing/or Negative Change in Any Domain	% of Subjects Changing in 1–2 Domains	% Changing in 3–5 Domains
Learning difficulties	70	3.75%	43.7%	40%
Mental illness	149	8.72%	37.58%	53.69%
Orthopedic	93	4.3%	33.69%	61.95%
Respiratory disease	76	12%	44%	44%
Acquired neurology stroke	45	9.52%	42.85%	47.62%
Frail elderly (multifactorial)	24	8.3%	33.33%	58.3%

PHYSIOTHERAPY

A total of 13,348 patients, representing a broad range of etiologies and impairments, were included in the study. These results were gathered from eight collaborating physiotherapy departments with involvement of 52 physiotherapists. The departments included those in District General Hospitals, specialist rehabilitation units, mental illness units, and community care. Of the 13,348 patients, 697 patients were noted to have more than one impairment and 534 patients had a carer well-being score noted.

Combined Scores for All Client Groups—Physiotherapy

The average number of contacts for all the patients in this study were 6.35 over an average duration of 1.65 months. The average start, change, and finish scores for all 13,348 patients from a broad range of etiologies and with widely varying impairments are presented in Table 4–6. Substantial gains are seen in the areas of impairment and disability with less marked changes in the areas of handicap and well-being.

Table 4–6. Average start, change, and finish scores for each domain—Physiotherapy (N = 13,348).

	F1	D	H	PWB	CWB (N = 534)
Start	2.8	2.95	3.65	4.1	3.7
Change	1	1.05	0.55	0.35	0.35
Finish	3.8	4.05	4.25	4.45	4.05

In such a heterogeneous group of patients one would expect that some patients will deteriorate in some domains whereas others may make great gains. Table 4–7 identifies the percentage of patients with the amount of change, thus 3% of patients deteriorated in their impairment, 2.8% deteriorated in their disability, and 2.5% in handicap, 26.8% of patients showed no change in their impairment, 28.5% of patients showed no change on disability, and just under half of the patients (46.4%) showed no change on handicap, with more than half (62%) showing no change on well-being. Between 38% and 40% of patients showed gains of between .5 and 1 point on the domains of impairment, disability, and handicap.

Table 4–7. Percentage of patients with change amount: Physiotherapy (N = 13,348).

	F1	**D**	**H**	**PWB**	**CWB**
Negative	3	2.8	2.5	2.6	2.6
None	26.8	28.5	46.4	62	54.3
0.6–1	40	37.3	38	27.8	26.4
1.6–2	20.7	18.3	10.4	5.6	4.6
2.6–3	7.5	7.8	2	1.3	1.6
3.6–5	1.7	5.1	0.3	0.4	4.3

Table 4–8. reflects the numbers of patients who changed in more than one domain. A total of 1,570 patients did not change in any domain over this 9-month period, but it must be remembered that some of these patients had not completed their period of treatment and some would have been in a long-term maintenance program. This table illustrates that 35% of patients changed in one or two domains but over half (51.28%) changed in three or more domains.

Table 4–8. Number of domain changes: Physiotherapy (N = 13348).

None	**1**	**2**	**3**	**4**	**5**
1570	1676	3247	3557	3127	152

Client-Specific Group Results—Physiotherapy

The average start, change, and finish scores with the percentage change for different etiological groups for patients who have been through an episode of physiotherapy care are illustrated in Table 4–9. Again the percentage change is dependent on the initial score as explained in the section on occupational therapy. For example a small change from a low score, has a higher percentage improvement than a small change from a higher base score. Thus the percentage change for this study has been calculated by subtracting the start score from the finish score and dividing by the start score and then multiplying by 100. Not all patients had a carer involved in their treatment program. For some patient groups the numbers of carer well-being scores that were collected were extremely low and caution should be taken when drawing any conclusions on the basis of findings related to small samples.

High gains in both impairment and disability were shown in the areas of orthopedic-spinal surgery (impairment gain of 75%, disability gain of 102%); orthopedic-joint replacement (impairment gain of 108.3%, disability gain of 172%); and orthopedic-fracture/dislocation (impairment gain of 66.6%, disability gain of 90.2%). Low gains and negative changes in the area of disability were noted for patients with the etiologies of progressive neurological disease, for example, motor neurone disease (impairment gain of −12.1%, disability gain of 6.9%).

Table 4–9. Physiotherapy: Average start, change, and finish scores with percentage change for different etiological groups.

Disorder	Number of Subjects	Number with Carer Well-being Score	First Impairment			Disability/Activity			Handicap/Participation			Patient Well-being			Carer Well-being		
			S	C %	F	S	C %	F	S	C %	F	S	C %	F	S	C %	F
Chronic respiratory disease	179	23	2.6	0.4 / 17.3%	3.05	2.65	0.55 / 22.6%	3.25	2.8	0.4 / 14.2%	3.2	3.24	0.45 / 13.84%	3.7	4	−0.2 / −3.75%	3.85
Acute respiratory disease	302	2	2.5	0.75 / 30%	3.25	2.45	0.9 / 38.7%	3.4	2.5	0.7 / 30%	3.25	3.3	0.45 / 13.6%	3.74	3.5	1 / 28.5%	4.5
Incontinence associated with obstetrics and gynecology	126	2	3.2	0.85 / 26.5%	4.05	3.4	0.9 / 27.9%	4.35	3.95	0.5 / 13.9%	4.5	4.1	0.55 / 13.4%	4.65	2.5	2.5 / 100%	5
Obstetrics and gynecology other than incontinence	346	2	3.8	0.55 / 15.8%	4.4	4.2	0.55 / 13.1%	4.75	3.8	0.65 / 17.1%	4.45	3.9	0.8 / 20.5%	4.7	1.5	1 / 66%	2.5
Cardiovascular disorder Myocardial infarction	29	0	2.75	0.75 / 27.2%	3.55	3.05	0.8 / 26.2%	3.85	3.25	0.6 / 18.5%	3.9	3.95	0.05 / 1.3%	4.05	—	—	—
Orthopedic spinal surgery	110	1	2.2	1.65 / 75%	3.9	2.05	2.1 / 102%	4.2	3.5	0.8 / 22.8%	4.35	4.2	0.4 / 9.5%	4.65	3	0 / —	3
Neurosurgery spinal surgery	76	1	2.45	1.4 / 57%	3.85	2.4	1.6 / 66.7%	4.05	3.45	0.8 / 23.2%	4.25	4.05	0.55 / 13.6%	4.6	5	0 / —	5
Spinal dysfunction Low back pain	1,548	12	2.95	1.1 / 37.3%	4.05	3.3	1.05 / 31.8%	4.35	4.05	0.55 / 13.6%	4.6	4.5	0.25 / 6.6%	4.8	3.55	0.45 / 12.6%	4
Spinal dysfunction Other	1,284	2	2.9	1.2 / 43.1%	4.15	3.3	1.1 / 33.3%	4.4	4.15	0.55 / 13.2%	4.7	4.5	0.3 / 7.7%	4.85	1.5	2.5 / 166%	4

continued

38

Table 4-9. (*continued*)

Disorder	Number of Subjects	Number with Carer Well-being Score	First Impairment S	First Impairment C %	First Impairment F	Disability/ Activity S	Disability/ Activity C %	Disability/ Activity F	Handicap/ Participation S	Handicap/ Participation C %	Handicap/ Participation F	Patient Well-being S	Patient Well-being C %	Patient Well-being F	Carer Well-being S	Carer Well-being C %	Carer Well-being F
Orthopedic Fracture/ dislocation	1,351	28	2.1	1.4 66.6%	3.5	2.05	1.85 90.2%	3.9	3.4	0.75 22%	4.15	4.1	0.4 9.7%	4.5	3.55	0.85 23.9%	4.4
Orthopedic Joint replacement	529	15	1.8	108.3%	3.8	1.45	2.5 172%	3.95	3.3	0.95 28.8%	4.25	4.05	0.6 14.8%	4.65	4.4	0.45 10.2%	4.85
Musculoskeletal Osteoarthritis	679	19	2.95	0.7 25.4%	3.7	3.35	0.6 19.4%	4	3.85	0.4 10.4%	4.25	4.25	0.3 7.0%	4.55	3.7	-0.15 -2.7%	3.6
Musculoskeletal Other	3,485	62	3.1	1.05 35.5%	4.2	3.45	0.95 29%	4.45	4.2	0.45 11.9%	4.7	4.6	0.2 4.3%	4.8	3.5	0.65 18.6%	4.2
Acquired neurological Head injury	29	3	2.9	0.6 20.6%	3.55	2.4	0.85 35.4%	3.25	2.35	0.8 34%	3.2	2.95	0.4 13.4%	3.4	3.65	0.15 4.1%	3.8
Acquired neurological CVA	281	32	2.55	0.4 15.7%	2.95	2.25	0.65 28.9%	2.95	2.2	0.6 27.3%	2.8	2.95	0.4 13.5%	3.4	3.75	0.1 2.9%	3.85
Progressive neurological disease—M.S.	25	3	2.6	0.25 9.6%	2.9	2.65	0.45 17%	3.15	2.95	0.4 13.5%	3.4	3.75	0.2 5.3%	3.95	3.3	0.3 9.0%	3.65
Progressive neurological disease—P.D.	34	4	2.7	0.35 13%	3.1	2.7	0.55 20.4%	3.25	2.5	0.5 20%	3.05	3.05	0.4 13.1%	3.45	3	0.85 28.3%	3.85
Progressive neurological disease—MND	13	4	2.05	-0.25 -12.1%	1.8	2.15	0.15 6.9%	2.3	2.3	-0.2 -8.6%	2.1	2.65	0.1 3.8%	2.8	4.25	0.25 5.9%	4.5
Senile dementia	35	5	2.9	0.25 8.6%	3.15	2.75	0.2 7.3%	3	1.95	0.25 12.8%	2.2	2.2	0.15 6.8%	2.4	3.75	0.4 10.6%	4.15

Musculoskeletal JCA	70	10	3	0.8 26.7%	3.8	3.4	0.65 19.1%	4.05	3.65	0.6 16.4%	4.3	3.85	0.55 14.3%	4.45	4.05	0.3 7.4%	4.4
Congenital Cerebral palsy children	96	77	2.15	0.15 7%	2.35	2.3	0.2 8.7%	2.55	2.65	0.2 7.5%	2.85	2.95	0.25 8.5%	3.25	3.65	0.05 1.4%	3.75
Congenital neurological deficit (not CP)	53	25	2.65	0.2 7.5%	2.85	2.3	0.35 15.2%	2.7	2.6	0.35 13.5%	3	3.25	0.3 9.2%	3.6	3.45	0.45 13.0%	3.95

Note: S = Start, C = Change, F = Finish

Cerebral Palsy children (impairment gain of 7%, disability gain of 8.7%). Some of these low change scores are related to the underlying nature of the pathology and some to the fact that the study was carried over a 9-month period. It would be less likely for substantial changes to be found in patients with, for example, congenital cerebral palsy, over such a short period of time.

Patient well-being was particularly improved in the area of obstetrics and gynecology (20.5% gain) but showed little change in patients with motor neurone disease (3.8% gain).

Patients with senile dementia had particularly compromised handicap/participation scores at the start of treatment (1.95%), but this improved over the period of treatment to show a gain of 12.8%. Patients with many of the musculoskeletal and spinal disorders did not show that their handicap/participation scores were specifically affected by their disorder. Of this group those who had undergone spinal orthopedic surgery were most compromised and made greatest gains (22.8%).

As with the results in occupational therapists, we were again surprised to find that so few patients had carer well-being scores. With some groups this is because a carer was not identifiable or not available to participate in treatment, but with other client groups it is suspected that a therapist did not feel that it was appropriate or necessary to collect information related to this domain. Of the groups with a sufficient number of carer well-being scores, those with musculoskeletal disorders showed the best gains (18.6%). A total of 25 carers of persons with congenital neurological deficit (children) showed a gain of 13% in their well-being score over this short period of time, whereas 77 carers of children with cerebral palsy showed a gain of 1.4% over the same period.

The clinical trial was conducted to establish whether this approach of collecting outcome measures was practical as well as whether it reflected the changes one would expect. The data presented here appear to have face validity, reflecting that patients with chronic and severe conditions make smaller gains in some areas than those with more transient or acute conditions. Furthermore, some client groups would be expected to change more dramatically in the area of disability, participation, or well-being but their impairment may be more resistant to change due to the underlying nature of the condition. The clinical trial seems to support the assertion that the Therapy Outcome Measure can reflect the expected course of a disorder.

The therapists involved in the trial reported that they became quicker in being able to gather information and they did not find it overly time consuming or stressful. The majority of therapists reported that they were able to complete an outcome rating in less than 3 minutes once they became familiar with the scales and the form.

Revised

References

Cohen, J. (1968). Weighted Kappa: nominal scale agreement with provision for scaled disagreement or partial credit. *Psychological Bulletin, 70*, 213–220.

Cowley, A. J., Fullwood, L. J., Muller, A. F., Stainer, K., Skene, A. M., & Hampton, J. R. (1991). Exercise capability in heart failure: Is cardiac output important after all. *Lancet, 33*, 771–773.

Enderby, P., (1992). Outcome measures in speech therapy: impairment, disability, handicap and distress. *Health Trends. 24*(2), 61–64.

Enderby, P. & John, A. (1997). *Therapy outcome measures: Speech-language pathology.* San Diego: Singular Publishing Group.

Frattali, C. (1991, September). Professional practices perspective. *Asha, 12.*

Fugl-Meyer, A. R., Branholm, I. B., & Fugl-Meyer, K. S. (1991). Happiness and domain specific life satisfaction in adult northern Swedes. *Clinical Rehabilitation, 5*, 25–33.

Gamiats, T. G., Palinkas, L. A., & Kaplan. R. (1992). Comparison of quality of wellbeing scale and functional status index in patients with atrial fibrillation. *Medical Care, 30*, 958–964.

Guildford, J. P. (1954). *Psychometric methods.* New York: McGraw-Hill.

Langton-Hewer, R. (1990). Outcome measures in stroke. A British view. *Stroke, 21*(Suppl II), 11–52.

Long, A. F. (1996). The user perspective in outcome measure: An overview of the issues. *Outcomes Briefings, 8.*

Maclure, M., Willett, W. C. (1987). Misinterpretation and misuse of the Kappa statistic. *American Journal of Epidemilogy. 126*, 161–169.

McCrae, R. R., & Costa, P. T. (1986). Personality, coping and coping effectiveness in an adult sample. *Journal of Personality, 2*, 285–405.

McKenna, S. P., Hunt, S. M., & Tennant, A. (1993). The development of a patient completed index of distress from the Nottingham Health Profile: A new measure for use in cost utility studies. *British Journal of Medical Economics, 6*, 13–24.

Paterson, C. (1996). Measuring outcomes in primary care: A patient generated measure. MYMOP compared with SF36 Health Survey. *British Medical Journal, 312*, 106–1020.

Rosser, R. M. (1976). Recent studies using a global approach to measuring illness. *Medical Care, 14*(Suppl. 5), 138–147.

Stephen, D., & Hetu, R. (1992). Impairment disability and handicap in audiology; towards a consensus. *Audiology*, 1–15.

Streiner, D. L., & Norman, G. R. (1989). *Health measurement scales: A practical guide to their development and use* (chap. 8). New York: Oxford University Press.

Ustun, B. (1997). News on the ICIDH. Centre for Standisation of Informatics in Health Care; *Newsletter, 4*, 2–7.

Whiteneck, S., Charlifue, S. W., Gerhart, K. A., Overholson, J. D., & Richardson, N. (1992). Quantifying handicap: A new measure of a long-term rehabilitation outcome. *Archives of Physical Medicine and Rehabilitation, 73*, 519–525.

Williams, S. J., & Bury, M. R. (1989). "Breathtaking" the consequence of chronic respiratory disorder. *International Disability Studies, 11*, 114–120.

Wilkin, J., Hallam, L., & Doggett, M. (1992). *Measures of need and outcome for primary health care.* Oxford: Oxford University Press.

Wood, P. H. (1980). The language of disablement: A glossary relating to disease and its consequences. *International Rehabilitation Medicine, 2*, 86–92.

Wood, P. H. N., & Badley, E. M. (1978). An epidemiological appraisal of disablement. In A. E. Bennett (Ed.), *Recent advances in community medicine.* Edinburgh: Churchill Livingstone.

Appendix 1

Core Scale

Impairment

0   The most severe presentation of this impairment.
1   Severe presentation of this impairment.
2   Severe/moderate presentation.
3   Moderate presentation.
4   Just below normal/mild presentation.
5   No impairment.

Disability

0   Totally dependent/unable to function.
1   Assists/cooperates but burden of task/achievement falls on professional or carer.
2   Can undertake some part of task but needs a high level of support to complete.
3   Can undertake task/function in familiar situation but requires some verbal/physical assistance.
4   Requires some minor assistance occasionally or extra time to complete task.
5   Independent/able to function.

Handicap

0   No autonomy, isolated, no social/family role.
1   Very limited choices, contact mainly with professionals, no social or family role, little control over life.
2   Some integration, value, and autonomy in one setting.
3   Integrated, valued, and autonomous in limited number of settings.
4   Occasionally some restriction in autonomy, integration, or role.
5   Integrated, valued, occupies appropriate role.

Distress/Well-Being

0   High and constant levels of concern/anger/severe depression or apathy, unable to express or control emotions appropriately.
1   Moderate concern, becomes concerned easily, requires constant reassurance/support, needs clear/tight limits and structure, loses emotional control easily.
2   Concern in unfamiliar situation, frequent emotional encouragement and support required.
3   Controls emotions with assistance, emotionally dependent on some occasions, vulnerable to change in routine etc., spontaneously uses methods to assist emotional control.
4   Able to control feelings in most situations, generally well adjusted/stable (most of the time/most situations), occasional emotional support/encouragement needed.
5   Well adjusted, stable, and able to cope with most situations, opportunity to self-analyze, accepts and understands own limitations.

Appendix 2

Detailed Scales: Physiotherapy/Occupational Therapy/Nursing Rehabilitation[1]

[1]If patient has more than one impairment (e.g., Head Injury and Cognitive Disorder), reflect the primary impairment code in Imp 1 and the secondary impairment in Imp 2.

ANXIETY

Impairment

0   Continual demonstration of global severe symptoms with no relief.

1   Severe anxiety/stress symptoms demonstrated most of the time but sometimes there are circumstances where partial relief is experienced.

2   Some situations/times when anxiety/stress is severe or moderate anxiety/stress frequently experienced (daily) but there are periods when anxiety is not a problem.

3   Anxiety/stress occasionally severe (weekly); can manage stress on some occasions but may need prompting and support with strategies.

4   Anxiety/stress levels easily aroused but copes when strategies in place, very occasional difficulties.

5   Normal response in stressful situations.

Disability

0   Physically dependent for all functional tasks. No self-care skills.

1   Dependent for most tasks but will cooperate. Physical assistance required frequently. Carer undertaking burden of tasks.

2   Most tasks, needs verbal and physical prompts to initiate.

3   Some physical/verbal support and encouragement to complete some tasks but initiates appropriately.

4   Occasional verbal encouragement needed and support or extra time required for specific tasks.

5   Independent in all areas.

Handicap

0   Social isolation, no interaction, very little quality of life, no autonomy. Lack of self-esteem, or self-worth. Unable to exercise choice.

1   Very limited control of immediate environment, poor self-esteem, minimal autonomy with immediate carers only. Unable to exercise choice.

2   Marked loss or change of role, e.g., nonintegrated recreation, nonintegrated education/occupation, limited access to different community environments, autonomy in immediate environment. Limited choices available.

3   Has a role in some surroundings but this may be diminished or changed, e.g., unable to fulfill usual work or sport activities. Some limited access to general environment facilities, has autonomy within domicile and other familiar environments but limited choice and control in a number of situations.

4   Some difficulty with sustaining expected roles (work, family, leisure), occasional restricted access to activities, reduced option for lifestyle. Has reduced choice and control in some situations.

5   Integrated and able to maintain expected different roles in society. Valued by others. Exercises choice and autonomy.

Distress/Well-Being

0   High and constant levels of concern/anger/severe depression or apathy, unable to express or control emotions appropriately.

1   Moderate concern, becomes concerned easily, requires constant reassurance/support, needs clear/tight limits and structure, loses emotional control easily.

2   Concern in unfamiliar situations, frequent emotional encouragement and support required.

3   Controls emotions with assistance, emotionally dependent on some occasions, vulnerable to change in routine, etc., spontaneously uses methods to assist emotional control.

4   Able to control feelings in most situations, generally well adjusted/stable (most of the time/most situations), occasional emotional support/encouragement needed.

5   Well adjusted, stable and able to cope emotionally with most situations, good insight, accepts and understands own limitations.

CARDIAC REHABILITATION

Impairment

0   Severe uncontrolled angina, uncontrolled cardiac failure.

1   Moderate control of cardiac function with multiple drug therapy.

2   Cardiac function and angina mostly controlled with regular medication, at times not controlled.

3   Cardiac function and angina controlled with regular medication.

4   Cardiac function maintained with occasional or minimal medication.

5   Normal cardiac function.

Disability

0   Lacks functional ability, dependent due to severe chest pain/breathlessness/weakness/dizziness on minimal exertion, e.g., when being transferred from bed to chair.

1   Very limited functional ability, chest pain/breathlessness/weakness/dizziness limiting activities of daily living, e.g., washing, dressing, mobilizing to toilet.

2   Function limited by chest pain/breathlessness/weakness/dizziness, e.g., walking on level ground (100 yards) or one flight of stairs.

3   Moderate functional ability, chest pain/breathlessness/weakness/dizziness on moderate exertion, e.g., 1 minute each stage of 10 stage exercise circuit.

4   Mild effect on functional ability, some occasional reduction in complex tasks due to pain/breathlessness.

5   No functional disability-able to tackle normal activities.

Handicap

0   Social isolation, no interaction, very little quality of life, no autonomy. Lack of self-esteem, or self-worth. Unable to exercise choice.

1   Very limited control of immediate environment, mainly limited to one environment, poor self-esteem, minimal autonomy with immediate carers only. Unable to exercise choice.

2   Marked loss or change of role, e.g., nonintegrated recreation, nonintegrated education/occupation, limited access to different community environments, autonomy in immediate environment. Limited choices available.

3   Has a role in some surroundings but this may be diminished or changed, e.g., unable to fulfill usual work or sport activities. Some limited access to general environment facilities, has autonomy within domicile and other familiar environments but limited choice and control in number of situations.

4   Some difficulty with sustaining expected roles (work, family, leisure), occasional restricted access to activities, reduced option for lifestyle. Has reduced choice and control in some situations.

5   Integrated and able to maintain expected roles in society. Valued by others. Exercises choice and autonomy.

Distress/Well-Being

0   High and constant levels of concern/anxiety/severe depression or apathy; unable to express or control emotions appropriately.

1   Moderate concern, becomes concerned easily, requires constant reassurance/support, needs clear/tight limits and structure, loses emotional control easily.

2   Concern in unfamiliar situations, frequent emotional encouragement and support required.

3   Controls emotions with assistance, emotionally dependent on some occasions, vulnerable to change in routine, etc., spontaneously uses methods to assist emotional control.

4   Able to control feelings in most situations, generally well adjusted/stable (most of the time/most situations), occasional emotional support/encouragement needed.

5   Well adjusted, stable, and able to cope emotionally with most situations, good insight, accepts and understands own limitations.

CEREBRAL PALSY

Impairment

0   Severe abnormality of tone with total body involvement. Fixed or at risk of severe contractures and deformities. No voluntary movement. Severe sensory impairment.

1   Severe abnormality of tone with total body involvement. At risk of severe contractures and deformities. Minimal voluntary movement. Severe sensory impairment.

2   Moderate abnormality of tone with total body involvement or severe involvement of 2 limbs. At risk of contractures and deformities. Potential for voluntary movement. Moderate sensory impairment.

3   Moderate abnormality of tone with partial involvement or severe single limb involvement. Little risk of contractures or deformities. Impaired voluntary movement. Mild sensory impairment.

4   Mild abnormality of tone with no contractures and deformities. Mild impairment in voluntary movement. Minimal sensory impairment.

5   No impairment.

Disability

0   No purposeful active movement, totally dependent, requires full physical care and constant vigilant supervision. May have totally disruptive and uncooperative behavior. Totally dependent on skilled assistance.

1   Bed-chair-bound but unable to sit independently. Some very limited purposeful activity. Needs high level of assistance in most tasks. Some awareness, some effort and recognition to contribute to care. Dependent on skilled assistance.

2   Head and trunk control. Limited self-help skills. Initiates some aspects of ADL. Transfers with one, mobilizes with two. Requires physical and verbal prompting and supervision for most tasks and movements. Participating in care and engaging in some structured activity. Dependent on familiar assistant.

3   Transfers or walking requires supervision or help of one. Undertakes personal care in modified supported environment. Appropriately initiating activities, needs assistance or supervision with some unfamiliar or complex tasks. Initiates activities appropriately.

4   Carrying out personal care and tasks but is less efficient, clumsy, requires extra time or may need encouragement, uses prompts effectively. Minimal or occasional assistance required for some complex tasks.

5   Age appropriate independence. [1]

[1]Consider age appropriacy.

Handicap

0   Unable to be integrated into any age appropriate activities, no relationships, no autonomy, lack of self-esteem. Unable to exercise choice. Lacking role.

1   Very limited control of immediate environment, mainly limited to one environment, poor self-esteem, minimal autonomy with immediate carers only. Limited role.

2   Able to access very few educational/work and leisure facilities. Has autonomy for basic choices only. Valued roles in restricted environment with limited number of individuals.

3   Has a role in some surroundings but this may be diminished or changed, e.g., unable to fulfill usual education, work, or leisure activities. Some limited access to general environment facilities, has autonomy within domicile and other familiar environments. Fulfilling role in certain areas.

4   Integrated with support into wider social environment/school/community/leisure. Has a valued role. Can exercise choice and control, some reduction in options of lifestyle with reduction of choice and control in a few situations.

5   Integrated and able to maintain expected different roles in society. Valued by others. Exercises choice and autonomy.

Distress/Well-Being

0   High and constant levels of concern/anger/severe depression or apathy, unable to express or control emotions appropriately.

1   Moderate concern, becomes concerned easily, requires constant reassurance/support, needs clear/tight limits and structure, loses emotional control easily.

2   Concern in unfamiliar situation, frequent emotional encouragement and support required.

3   Controls emotions with assistance, emotionally dependent on some occasions, vulnerable to change in routine, etc., spontaneously uses methods to assist emotional control.

4   Able to control feelings in most situations, generally well adjusted/stable (most of the time/most situations), occasional emotional support/encouragement needed.

5   Well adjusted, stable, and able to cope emotionally with most situations, good insight, accepts and understands own limitations.

COGNITION

Impairment

0   Unresponsive to all stimuli. Does not recognize people, unable to learn, poor memory responses, frequent inappropriate responses.

1   Nonpurposeful random or fragmented responses. Occasionally responds to some simple commands; may respond to discomfort; responses may be severely delayed. Recognizes familiar people and routine tasks in context. Cooperates occasionally, attempts to learn simplest routines with maximal assistance.

2   Inconsistent reaction directly related to type of stimulus presented. Can attend but is highly distractible and unable to focus on a particular task. Memory is severely impaired; may perform previously learned task with structure but is unable to retain new information. Recognizes familiar people and tasks in most contexts, able to retain small amounts of information consistently. Occasionally responds appropriately.

3   Correct routine responses may be robot-like, appears oriented to setting, but insight, judgment, and problem solving poor. Memory variable—sometimes very good, learning more complex tasks, responds appropriately more frequently.

4   Able to recall and integrate past and recent events; shows carryover for new learning and needs no supervision when activities are learned, but has high level difficulties, for example, abstract reasoning, tolerance for stress, or judgment in unusual circumstances. Alert and able to learn-but needs occasional prompts and assistance, responds well in most situations.

5   No cognitive impairment. Alert, able to learn, responds appropriately.

Disability

0   Inability to recognize body functions and requirements. May have totally disruptive and uncooperative behavior. Totally dependent; requires full physical care and constant vigilant supervision.

1   Recognizes bodily requirements and occasionally initiates activity but requires high level of assistance in most tasks.

2   Able to self-care and relate to others in protected environment but is dependent on constant verbal prompting and direction.

3   Needs occasional verbal prompting to initiate activity. Able to operate without supervision for short periods, able to have some independence with encouragement, independent in familiar surroundings only.

4   Able to live independently with some occasional support, requires extra time, encouragement. Assistance required with unfamiliar tasks.

5   Age appropriate independence.

Handicap

0   Social isolation, no interaction, very little quality of life, no autonomy. Lack of self-esteem, or self-worth. Unable to exercise choice.

1   Very limited control of immediate environment, poor self-esteem, minimal autonomy with immediate carers only. Unable to exercise choice.

2   Marked loss or change of role, e.g., nonintegrated recreation, nonintegrated education/occupation, limited access to different community environments, autonomy in immediate environment. Limited choices available.

3   Has a role in some surroundings but this may be diminished or changed, e.g., unable to fulfill usual work or sport activities. Some limited access to general environment facilities, has autonomy within domicile and other familiar environments but limited choice and control in a number of situations.

4   Some difficulty with sustaining expected roles (work, family, leisure), occasional restricted access to activities, reduced option for lifestyle. Has reduced choice and control in some situations.

5   Integrated and able to maintain expected different roles in society. Valued by others. Exercises choice and autonomy.

Distress/Well-Being

0   High and constant levels of concern/anger/severe depression or apathy, unable to express or control emotions appropriately.

1   Moderate concern, becomes concerned easily, requires constant reassurance/support, needs clear/tight limits and structure, loses emotional control easily.

2   Concern in unfamiliar situations, frequent emotional encouragement and support required.

3   Controls emotions with assistance, emotionally dependent on some occasions, vulnerable to change in routine, etc., spontaneously uses methods to assist emotional control.

4   Able to control feelings in most situations, generally well adjusted/stable (most of the time/most situations), occasional emotional support/encouragement needed.

5   Well adjusted, stable, and able to cope emotionally with most situations, good insight, accepts and understands own limitations.

COMPLEX AND MULTIPLE DIFFICULTY

Impairment (as appropriate to age)

0   No purposeful active movement, severe abnormality of muscle tone and patterns of movement, sensory loss, may have severe fixed deformities. Presence of pathological reflexes.
Total body involvement.

1   Grossly abnormal muscle tone, occasionally some voluntary movement toward stimulus,
some contractures, some pathological reflexes, sensory loss, severely restricted range of
movement. Total body involvement.

2   Altered muscle tone, some purposeful active movement/abnormal reflex activity/primitive
reflexes. Some joint contractures, marked sensory impairment. May have involvement of
most body parts but some not impaired, e.g., hemiplegia and poor trunk control.

3   Some useful strength, but abnormal muscle tone, coordinates movement without accuracy,
requires large stable base and low center of gravity, moderate sensory loss. May have
involvement of two body parts.

4   Slight abnormality of strength, muscle tone, range of movement, minimal involuntary movements. Slightly impaired neurology with mild weakness or incoordination. May have severe
involvement of one body part (e.g., one limb).

5   Age appropriate tone, strength, range of movement, and coordination.

Disability (as appropriate to age)

0   No purposeful active movement, totally dependent, requires full physical care and constant
vigilant supervision. May have totally disruptive and uncooperative behavior. Dependent on
skilled assistance.

1   Bed-chair-bound but unable to sit independently. Some very limited purposeful activity.
Needs high level of assistance in all tasks. Some awareness, some effort and recognition to
contribute to care. Dependent on skilled assistance.

2   Head and trunk control. Limited self-help skills. Initiates some aspects of ADL. Transfers
with one, mobilizes with two. Requires physical and verbal prompting and supervision for
most tasks and movements. Participating in care and engaging in some structured activity.
Dependent on familiar assistance.

3   Transfers or walking require supervision or help of one. Undertakes personal care in modified supported environment. Appropriately initiating activities, needs assistance or supervision with unfamiliar or complex tasks. Initiates activities appropriately.

4   Carrying out personal care and tasks but is less efficient, clumsy, requires extra time, or may
need encouragement, uses memory prompts and other aids effectively. Minimal or occasional assistance required for some complex or unfamiliar tasks.

5   Age appropriate independence.

Handicap (as appropriate to age)

0   Social isolation, no interaction, very little quality of life, no autonomy. Lack of self-esteem, or self-worth. Unable to exercise choice.

1   Very limited control of immediate environment, poor self-esteem, minimal autonomy with immediate carers only. Unable to exercise choice.

2   Marked loss or change of role, e.g., nonintegrated recreation, nonintegrated education/occupation, limited access to different community environments, autonomy in immediate environment. Limited choices available.

3   Has a role in some surroundings but this may be diminished or changed, e.g., unable to fulfill usual work or sport activities. Some limited access to general environment facilities, has autonomy within domicile and other familiar environments but limited choice and control in a number of situations.

4   Some difficulty with sustaining expected roles (work, family, leisure), occasional restricted access to activities, reduced option for lifestyle. Has reduced choice and control in some situations.

5   Integrated and able to maintain expected different roles in society. Valued by others. Exercises choice and autonomy.

Distress/Well-Being (as appropriate to age)

0   High and constant levels of concern/anger/severe depression or apathy, unable to express or control emotions appropriately.

1   Moderate concern, becomes concerned easily, requires constant reassurance/support, needs clear/tight limits and structure, loses emotional control easily.

2   Concern in unfamiliar situations, frequent emotional encouragement and support required.

3   Controls emotions with assistance, emotionally dependent on some occasions, vulnerable to change in routine, etc., spontaneously uses methods to assist emotional control.

4   Able to control feelings in most situations, generally well adjusted/stable (most of the time/most situations), occasional emotional support/encouragement needed.

5   Well adjusted, stable, and able to cope emotionally with most situations, good insight, accepts and understands own limitations.

DYSPRAXIA
(Children with Developmental Coordination Difficulties)

Impairment (as appropriate to age)

0   Profound problems evident in all areas of sensory-motor development including vestibular, sensory processing and modulation, movement and task planning and organization, balance and coordination. Also perceptual and ideational difficulties. Severe generalized/motor impairment. Very limited attention to tasks. Examples of test scores 2.5 years behind actual age, first percentile, at or below 55 on a standard score.

1   Severe problems usually involving all areas as indicated above, or may involve severe problems in two or more areas or one profound overriding problem, e.g., severe sensory defensiveness or motor impairment. Examples of test scores on the second percentile, a 65 on a standard score.

2   Severe/moderate impairment. Severe to moderate problems in some areas, may involve one severe overriding area, for example, gross or fine motor skills, perception, coordination, handwriting, or movement planning. Examples of test scores on the fifth percentile, a delay of 2 to 2.5 years, at or below 73 on a standard score.

3   Moderate impairment. Moderate problems in some areas and/or specific moderate problems in one area, such as motor skills, organization, concentration, writing, or perception. Examples of test scores at or below 77 on a standard score on the seventh percentile, a lag of around 1.6 to 2 years.

4   Mild impairment. Mild problems in one or more areas involving fine or gross motor skills, perception, coordination, attention, praxis. Examples of test scores at or below 85 on a standard score, sixteenth percentile, a lag of over 1 year.

5   Age appropriate motor and perceptual development in all areas.

Disability (as appropriate to age)

0   Unable to function independently in any way. Unable to perform any activity without skilled and continual assistance, specialized equipment, supervision, or simplification.

1   Occasionally able to perform some simple/automatic activities independently, or to perform some parts of some tasks alone. Minimal function with maximum assistance.

2   Able to perform basic simple tasks or parts of more complex tasks. Works better with a familiar adult or family member, but lacks confidence in unfamiliar situations. Difficulty learning new skills or transferring them to different situations. Verbal prompts help.

3   Consistently able to perform simple tasks or parts of more complex ones without help. Can occasionally attempt new tasks building on existing skills. Needs help for some activities, or extra time, or tasks to be broken down or simplified. Verbal prompting may be needed.

4 Occasional difficulties experienced in certain situations or with certain activities. May require extra time to complete tasks. Occasional verbal prompts.

5 Functions well in all situations and is fully independent at an age appropriate level.

Handicap (as appropriate to age)

0 Unable to be integrated into any age appropriate activities, no relationships, no autonomy, lack of self-esteem. Unable to exercise choice. Lacking role.

1 Very limited control of immediate environment, mainly limited to one environment, poor self-esteem, minimal autonomy with immediate carers only. Limited role.

2 Able to access very few educational/work and leisure facilities. Has autonomy for basic choices only. Valued roles in restricted environment with limited number of individuals.

3 Has a role in some surroundings but this may be diminished or changed, e.g., unable to fulfill usual education, work, or leisure activities. Some limited access to general environment facilities, has autonomy within domicile and other familiar environments. Fulfilling role in certain areas.

4 Integrated with support into wider social environment/school/community/leisure. Has a valued role. Can exercise choice and control, some reduction in options of lifestyle with reduction of choice and control in a few situations.

5 Integrated and able to maintain expected different roles in society. Valued by others. Exercises choice and autonomy.

Distress/Well-Being

0 High and constant levels of concern/anger/severe depression or apathy, unable to express or control emotions appropriately.

1 Moderate concern, becomes concerned easily, requires constant reassurance/support, needs clear/tight limits and structure, loses emotional control easily.

2 Concern in unfamiliar situation, frequent emotional encouragement and support required.

3 Controls emotions with assistance, emotionally dependent on some occasions, vulnerable to change in routine, etc., spontaneously uses methods to assist emotional control.

4 Able to control feelings in most situations, generally well adjusted/stable (most of the time/most situations), occasional emotional support/encouragement needed.

5 Well adjusted, stable, and able to cope emotionally with most situations, good insight, accepts and understands own limitations.

HEAD INJURY

Impairment

0 Inability to respond to external stimuli/gross loss of passive range of movement affecting multiple joints. Debilitated, minimal muscle power, multijoint contractures/swelling. Total flaccidity/severe spasticity. Severe continual involuntary movements. Total loss of righting and equilibrium reactions. Severe global symptoms.

1 Responsive but uncooperative, range of movement maximally restricted. Passive range of movement moderately restricted. Pain on passive movement. No standing balance. Unable to bear weight. Power 2. Minimal controlled voluntary movement. Severe sensory inattention. Low tone/moderate spasticity. Strong associated reactions. Severe degree of several signs and symptoms, e.g., dense hemiplegia poor trunk control and some perceptual deficit.

2 Range of movement moderately restricted. Pain on active movement. Poor static balance. Some controlled purposeful movement. Moderate to severe inattention. Moderate involuntary movement. Associated reactions occurring on preparation to movement. Power 3.

3 Some active participation, active range of movement with minimal restriction. Some associated reactions during movement. Purposeful but not necessarily accurate voluntary movement. Moderate sensory inattention. Minimal involuntary movement. Intermittent pain on active movement. Poor dynamic standing balance. Power 3 plus. May have one severe sign or symptom alone, e.g., dense hemiplegia or severe perceptual deficit or combination of milder signs or symptoms, e.g., mild hemiparesis with some sensory loss and occasional incontinence.

4 Slight/minimal abnormality of strength, muscle tone, range of movement. Power 4, difficulty with balance, purposeful accurate voluntary movements. May have abnormal speed of movement, slight uncoordination. Minimal associated reaction with efforts.

5 Age appropriate strength, range of movement and coordination. Normal tone and active movements.

Disability

0 No purposeful active movement, totally dependent, requires full physical care and constant vigilant supervision. May have totally disruptive and uncooperative behavior. Dependent on skilled assistance.

1 Bed-chair-bound but unable to sit independently. Some very limited purposeful activity. Needs high level of assistance in most tasks. Some awareness, some effort and recognition to contribute to care. Dependent on skilled assistance.

2 Head and trunk control. Limited self-help skills. Initiates some aspects of ADL. Transfers with one, mobilizes with two. Requires physical and verbal prompting and supervision for most tasks and movements. Participating in care and engaging in some structured activity. Dependent on familiar assistant.

3   Transfers or walking requires supervision or help of one. Undertakes personal care in modified supported environment. Appropriately initiating activities and needs assistance or supervision with some unfamiliar or complex tasks. Initiates activities appropriately.

4   Carrying out personal care and tasks but is less efficient (clumsy), requires extra time or may need encouragement, assistance with unfamiliar tasks. Minimal or occasional assistance required for some complex tasks.

5   Age appropriate independence.

Handicap

0   Social isolation, no interaction, very little quality of life, no autonomy. Lack of self-esteem, or self-worth. Unable to exercise choice.

1   Very limited control of immediate environment, poor self-esteem, minimal autonomy with immediate carers only. Unable to exercise choice.

2   Marked loss or change of role, e.g., nonintegrated recreation, nonintegrated education/occupation, limited access to different community environments, autonomy in immediate environment. Limited choices available.

3   Has a role in some surroundings but this may be diminished or changed, e.g., unable to fulfill usual work or sport activities. Some limited access to general environment facilities, has autonomy within domicile and other familiar environments but limited choice and control in number of situations.

4   Some difficulty with sustaining expected roles (work, family, leisure), occasional restricted access to activities, reduced option for lifestyle. Has reduced choice and control in some situations.

5   Integrated and able to maintain expected different roles in society. Valued by others. Exercises choice and autonomy.

Distress/Well-Being

0   High and constant levels of concern/anger/severe depression or apathy, unable to express or control emotions appropriately.

1   Moderate concern, becomes concerned easily, requires constant reassurance/support, needs clear/tight limits and structure, loses emotional control easily.

2   Concern in unfamiliar situations, frequent emotional encouragement and support required.

3   Controls emotions with assistance, emotionally dependent on some occasions, vulnerable to change in routine, etc., spontaneously uses methods to assist emotional control.

4   Able to control feelings in most situations, generally well adjusted/stable (most of the time/most situations), occasional emotional support/encouragement needed.

5   Well adjusted, stable, and able to cope emotionally with most situations, good insight, accepts and understands own limitations.

INCONTINENCE

Impairment

0   No muscle power; bladder/bowel instability; no sensation, severe bladder/bowel prolapse; severe pain.

1   Flicker of muscle contraction. Intermittent severe pain.

2   Weak muscle contraction/diminished sensation. Some moderate pain.

3   Evidence of instability. Muscle contraction but not maintained against gravity. Occasional pain.

4   Muscle contraction against gravity. No pain; minor degree of prolapse.

5   Full muscle power and tone/stable bladder and bowel; full sensation, no prolapse.

Disability

0   Total lack of voluntary control; inability to recognize the need for bowel/bladder evacuation. Constant use of pads.

1   Recognizing need to evacuate but inability to control.

2   Some ability to control bowel/bladder/frequency/urgency; ability to go out for short periods with pads/toilet availability.

3   Intermittent bowel problems/frequent stress incontinence/urgency.

4   Very occasional stress incontinence of urine.

5   Full bladder and bowel control.

Handicap

0   Social isolation, no interaction, very little quality of life, no autonomy. Lack of self-esteem or self-worth. Unable to exercise choice.

1   Very limited control of immediate environment, housebound, poor self-esteem, minimal autonomy with immediate carers only. Unable to exercise choice.

2   Marked loss or change of role, e.g., nonintegrated recreation, nonintegrated education/occupation, limited access to different community environments, autonomy in immediate environment. Limited choices available.

3   Has a role in some surroundings but this may be diminished or changed, e.g., unable to fulfill usual work or sport activities. Some limited access to general environment facilities, has autonomy within domicile and other familiar environments but limited choice and control in number of situations.

4   Some difficulty with sustaining expected roles (work, family, leisure), occasional restricted access to activities, reduced option for lifestyle. Has reduced choice and control in some situations.

5   Integrated and able to maintain expected different roles in society. Valued by others. Exercises choice and autonomy.

Distress/Well-Being

0   High and constant levels of concern/anger/severe depression or apathy, unable to express or control emotions appropriately.

1   Moderate concern, becomes concerned easily, requires constant reassurance/support, needs clear/tight limits and structure, loses emotional control easily.

2   Concern in unfamiliar situations, frequent emotional encouragement and support required.

3   Controls emotions with assistance, emotionally dependent on some occasions, vulnerable to change in routine, etc., spontaneously uses methods to assist emotional control.

4   Able to control feelings in most situations, generally well adjusted/stable (most of the time/most situations), occasional emotional support/encouragement needed.

5   Well adjusted, stable, and able to cope emotionally with most situations, good insight, accepts and understands own limitations.

LEARNING DIFFICULTIES/MENTAL HANDICAP

Impairment

0 No active movement, severe abnormality of muscle tone and patterns of movement. May have abnormal sensory loss, severe fixed deformities, severe respiratory difficulties. Presence of pathological reflexes.

1 Grossly abnormal muscle tone, occasionally some voluntary movement toward stimulus, some contractures, some pathological reflexes, some sensory loss, severely restricted range of movement, frequent respiratory difficulties.

2 Altered muscle tone, some controlled purposeful active movement. Some abnormal primitive reflexes. Some joint contractures, moderate sensory impairment.

3 Useful strength, but abnormal muscle tone, coordinates movement but without accuracy, requires large stable base and low center of gravity, moderate sensory loss.

4 Slight abnormality of strength, muscle tone, range of movement; minimal involuntary movements. Slightly impaired neurology with mild weakness or uncoordination.

5 Age appropriate tone, strength, range of movement and coordination.

Disability

0 No purposeful active movement, totally dependent, requires full physical care and constant vigilant supervision. May have totally disruptive and uncooperative behavior. Dependent on skilled assistance.

1 Bed-chair-bound but unable to sit independently. Some very limited purposeful activity. Needs high level of assistance in most tasks. Some awareness, some effort and recognition to contribute to care. Dependent on skilled assistance.

2 Head and trunk control. Limited self-help skills. Initiates some aspects of ADL. Transfers with one, mobilizes with two. Requires physical and verbal prompting and supervision for most tasks and movements. Participating in care and engaging in some structured activity. Dependent on familiar assistance.

3 Transfers or walking require supervision or help of one. Undertakes personal care in modified supported environment. Appropriately initiating activities and needs assistance or supervision with some unfamiliar or complex tasks. Initiates activities appropriately.

4 Carrying out personal care and tasks but is less efficient (clumsy), requires extra time, or may need encouragement. Uses memory prompts or other aids effectively. Minimal or occasional assistance required for some complex or unfamiliar tasks.

5 Age appropriate independence.

Handicap

0   Social isolation, no interaction, very little quality of life, no autonomy. Lack of self-esteem, or self-worth. Unable to exercise choice.

1   Very limited control of immediate environment, poor self-esteem, minimal autonomy with immediate carers only. Unable to exercise choice.

2   Marked loss or change of role, e.g., nonintegrated recreation, nonintegrated education/occupation, limited access to different community environments, autonomy in immediate environment. Limited choices available.

3   Has a role in some surroundings but this may be diminished or changed, e.g., unable to fulfill usual work or sport activities. Some limited access to general environment facilities, has autonomy within domicile and other familiar environments but limited choice and control in number of situations.

4   Some difficulty with sustaining expected roles (work, family, leisure), occasional restricted access to activities, reduced option for lifestyle. Has reduced choice and control in some situations.

5   Integrated and able to maintain expected different roles in society. Valued by others. Exercises choice and autonomy.

Distress/Well-Being

0   High and constant levels of concern/anger/severe depression or apathy, unable to express or control emotions appropriately.

1   Moderate concern, becomes concerned easily, requires constant reassurance/support, needs clear/tight limits and structure, loses emotional control easily.

2   Concern in unfamiliar situations, frequent emotional encouragement and support required.

3   Controls emotions with assistance, emotionally dependent on some occasions, vulnerable to change in routine, etc., spontaneously uses methods to assist emotional control.

4   Able to control feelings in most situations, generally well adjusted/stable (most of the time/most situations), occasional emotional support/encouragement needed.

5   Well adjusted, stable, and able to cope emotionally with most situations, good insight, accepts and understands own limitations.

MENTAL HEALTH

Impairment

0   Catatonic, unresponsive; no volition, persistent/severe and wide range of thought disorders, fixed delusions, persistent visual, auditory, tactile hallucinations, persistent/severe disturbance of affect. Severe memory loss. No insight.

1   Severe thought disorder, auditory hallucinations frequent, variable disturbances of affect, little volition. Occasionally past memories recalled. Some automatic response. Apathetic, no motivation, no initiation. Recognizes own name and that of some individuals and situations. No insight into confusion.

2   Moderate thought disorder in duration, severity, frequency, some auditory hallucinations present, moderate disturbance of affect, moderate level of volition, some remote memory. Inappropriate responses to some stimuli. Occasional partial insight.

3   Evidence of some thought disorder, occasional evidence of auditory/visual hallucination, usually stable mood, volition intact. Some recent memory. Some insight. Attempting to express feeling and "sort things out." Orientated in regular surroundings, easily confused.

4   Very occasional evidence of some thought disorder in duration, severity, frequency, good level insight, usually stable mood, volition intact. Occasionally disturbed by new or occasional complex experiences. Short-term memory deficit. Can express feeling. Very occasional disorientation.

5   Well developed insight, high level volition, no evidence of thought disorder, delusion, hallucination. Appropriate memory. Orientated.

Disability

0   Inability to recognize body functions and requirements. May have totally disruptive and uncooperative behavior. Totally dependent, requires full physical care and constant vigilant supervision.

1   Recognizes some bodily requirements and occasionally initiates actively but requires high level of assistance and supervision in most tasks.

2   Able to cooperate in self-care and relate to others in protected environment but is dependent on verbal prompting to initiate and continue tasks. Requires some physical assistance.

3   Needs occasional verbal prompting to initiate movement/care, able to operate without supervision for short periods, able to have some independence with encouragement. Independent in familiar surroundings only.

4   Able to live independently with some occasional support, requires extra time, encouragement. Assistance occasionally required with unfamiliar tasks.

5 Age appropriate independence.

Handicap

0 Social isolation, no interaction, very little quality of life, no autonomy. Lack of self-esteem, or self-worth. Unable to exercise choice.

1 Very limited control of immediate environment. Poor self-esteem, minimal autonomy with immediate carers only. Unable to exercise choice.

2 Marked loss or change of role, e.g., nonintegrated recreation, nonintegrated education/occupation, limited access to different community environments, autonomy in immediate environment. Limited choices available.

3 Has a role in some surroundings but this may be diminished or changed, e.g., unable to fulfill usual work or sport activities. Some limited access to general environment facilities, has autonomy within domicile and other familiar environments but limited choice and control in a number of situations.

4 Some difficulty with sustaining expected roles (work, family, leisure), occasional restricted access to activities, reduced option for lifestyle. Has reduced choice and control in some situations.

5 Integrated and able to maintain expected different roles in society. Valued by others. Exercises choice and autonomy.

Distress/Well-Being

0 High and constant levels of concern/anger/severe depression or apathy, unable to express or control emotions appropriately.

1 Moderate concern, becomes concerned easily, requires constant reassurance/support, needs clear/tight limits and structure, loses emotional control easily.

2 Concern in unfamiliar situations, frequent emotional encouragement and support required.

3 Controls emotions with assistance, emotionally dependent on some occasions, vulnerable to change in routine, etc., spontaneously uses methods to assist emotional control.

4 Able to control feelings in most situations, generally well adjusted/stable (most of the time/most situations), occasional emotional support/encouragement needed.

5 Well adjusted, stable, and able to cope emotionally with most situations, good insight, accepts and understands own limitations.

MULTIFACTORIAL CONDITIONS
(e.g., complex physical disability, frail elderly)

Impairment

0   Inability to respond to external stimuli/gross loss of passive range of movement affecting multiple joints. Debilitated, minimal muscle power, multijoint contractures/swelling. Total flaccidity/severe spasticity. Severe continual involuntary movements. Total loss of righting and equilibrium reactions. Global severity of all symptoms.

1   Responsive but uncooperative, range of movement maximally restricted. Passive range of movement moderately restricted. Pain on passive movement. No standing balance. Unable to weight bear. Power 2. Minimal voluntary movement. Severe sensory inattention. Low tone/moderate spasticity. Strong associated reactions. Severe degree of several signs and symptoms, e.g., dense hemiplegia with some perceptual deficit. Responsive.

2   Active range of movement moderately restricted. Contractures in more than one joint. Pain on active movement. Poor static balance. Occasional purposeful movement. Moderate to severe inattention. Moderate involuntary movement. Associated reactions occurring on preparation to movement. Power 3. Aware and responsive.

3   Some active participation, active functional range of movement with minimal restriction. Intermittent pain on active movement. Poor dynamic standing balance. Some associated reactions during movement. Purposeful but not necessarily accurate voluntary movement. Moderate sensory inattention. Minimal involuntary movement. Power 3 plus. May have one severe sign or symptom alone, e.g., dense hemiplegia or severe perceptual deficit or combination of milder signs or symptoms, e.g., mild hemiparesis with some sensory loss and occasional incontinence.

4   Slight/minimal abnormality of strength, muscle tone, range of movement. Power 4, occasional difficulty with balance, purposeful accurate voluntary movements. May have abnormal speed of movement, slight incoordination. Minimal associated reaction with efforts. Mild occasional inattention.

5   Age appropriate strength, range of movement, and coordination. Normal tone and active movements.

Disability

0   No purposeful active movement, totally dependent, requires full physical care and constant vigilant supervision. May have totally disruptive and uncooperative behavior. Dependent on skilled assistance.

1   Bed-chair-bound but unable to sit independently. Some very limited purposeful activity. Needs high level of assistance in most tasks. Some awareness, some effort and recognition to contribute to care. Dependent on skilled assistance.

2   Head and trunk control. Limited self-help skills. Initiates some aspects of ADL. Transfers with one, mobilizes with two. Requires physical and verbal prompting and supervision for

most tasks and movements. Participating in care and engaging in some structured activity. Dependent on skilled assistance.

3   Transfers or walking requires supervision or help of one. Undertakes personal care in modified supported environment. Appropriately initiating activities and needs assistance or supervision with some unfamiliar or complex tasks. Initiates activities appropriately.

4   Carrying out personal care and tasks but is less efficient, clumsy, requires extra time or may need encouragement. Uses memory prompts effectively. Minimal or occasional assistance required for some complex tasks.

5   Age appropriate independence.

Handicap

0   Social isolation, no interaction, very little quality of life, no autonomy. Lack of self-esteem or self-worth. Unable to exercise choice.

1   Very limited control of immediate environment, poor self-esteem, minimal autonomy with immediate carers only. Unable to exercise choice.

2   Marked loss or change of role, e.g., nonintegrated recreation, nonintegrated education/occupation, limited access to different community environments, autonomy in immediate environment. Limited choices available.

3   Has a role in some surroundings but this may be diminished or changed, e.g., unable to fulfill usual work or sport activities. Some limited access to general environment facilities, has autonomy within domicile and other familiar environments but limited choice and control in a number of situations.

4   Some difficulty with sustaining expected roles (work, family, leisure), occasional restricted access to activities, reduced option for lifestyle. Has reduced choice and control in some situations.

5   Integrated and able to maintain expected different roles in society. Valued by others. Exercises choice and autonomy.

Distress/Well-Being

0   High and constant levels of concern/anger/severe depression or apathy, unable to express or control emotions appropriately.

1   Moderate concern, becomes concerned easily, requires constant reassurance/support, needs clear/tight limits and structure, loses emotional control easily.

2   Concern in unfamiliar situations, frequent emotional encouragement and support required.

3   Controls emotions with assistance, emotionally dependent on some occasions, vulnerable to change in routine, etc., spontaneously uses methods to assist emotional control.

4   Able to control feelings in most situations, generally well adjusted/stable (most of the time/most situations), occasional emotional support/encouragement needed.

5   Well adjusted, stable and able to cope emotionally with most situations, good insight, accepts and understands own limitations.

MUSCULO-SKELETAL

Impairment

0   Crippling, chronic, severe nonreversible deformity, severe inhibiting pain in several joints/parts of body. Severely limited range of movement and muscle power.

1   Severely restricted range of movement, partially reversible deformity, constant inhibiting pain/abnormal tone.

2   Moderate reversible deformity, restricted range of movement, redeemable muscle damage, inhibiting pain causing altered movement, moderate increased or decreased muscle tone. Poor exercise tolerance.

3   Correctable/slight deformity/slight increase or decrease in muscle tone, 60% range of movement and muscle power. Intermittent pain resulting in occasional altered practice. Some inhibiting pain. Moderate exercise tolerance.

4   Slightly reduced muscle power, 80% range of movement, slightly reduced tolerance, occasional discomfort. Good exercise tolerance.

5   Full range of movement and power. No pain, no abnormal muscle tone.

Disability

0   Immobile, totally dependent in all/any environments. Unable to participate in tasks.

1   Can transfer with maximal skilled physical assistance. Requires maximal assistance with all personal activities of daily living.

2   Requires regular assistance with activities of daily living; can undertake some tasks independently.

3   Personal activities of daily living/transfers requiring supervision and some occasional help from carer.

4   Independent in adapted environment, needs occasional assistance or extra time with complex or unfamiliar activities.

5   Age appropriate; independent in all environments.

Handicap

0   Social isolation, no interaction, very little quality of life, no autonomy. Lack of self-esteem, or self-worth. Unable to exercise choice.

1   Very limited control of immediate environment, housebound, poor self-esteem, minimal autonomy with immediate carers only. Unable to exercise choice.

2 Marked loss or change of role, e.g., nonintegrated recreation, nonintegrated education/occupation, limited access to different community environments, autonomy in immediate environment. Limited choices available.

3 Has a role in some surroundings but this may be diminished or changed, e.g., unable to fulfill usual work or sport activities. Some limited access to general environment facilities, has autonomy within domicile and other familiar environments but limited choice and control in a number of situations.

4 Some difficulty with sustaining expected roles (work, family, leisure), occasional restricted access to activities, reduced option for lifestyle. Has reduced choice and control in some situations. Some modification of work or sport activity.

5 Integrated and able to maintain expected different roles in society. Valued by others. Exercises choice and autonomy.

Distress/Well-Being

0 High and constant levels of concern/anger/severe depression or apathy, unable to express or control emotions appropriately.

1 Moderate concern, becomes concerned easily, requires constant reassurance/support, needs clear/tight limits and structure, loses emotional control easily.

2 Concern in unfamiliar situations, frequent emotional encouragement and support required.

3 Controls emotions with assistance, emotionally dependent on some occasions, vulnerable to change in routine, etc., spontaneously uses methods to assist emotional control.

4 Able to control feelings in most situations, generally well adjusted/stable (most of the time/most situations), occasional emotional support/encouragement needed.

5 Well adjusted, stable and able to cope emotionally with most situations, good insight, accepts and understands own limitations.

NEUROLOGICAL DISORDERS
(including Progressive Neurological Disorders)

Impairment

0 No volitional movement. Total flaccidity/severe spasticity. Total sensory inattention. Severe continual involuntary movement. Total loss of righting plus equilibrium reactions. Severe global symptoms. May be primarily bed-bound.

1 Severe loss of motor or sensory function. All limbs and trunk affected. Occasional minimal voluntary movements. Severe sensory inattention. Moderate to severe involuntary movements.

2 Frequent voluntary movements. General associated reactions occurring on preparation to movement. Moderate to severe inattention. Moderate involuntary movement.

3 Severe abnormal tone in specific muscle groups or moderate impairment of tone globally. Specific associated reactions during preparation to move. Purposeful and controlled but not necessarily accurate or strong voluntary movement. Moderate sensory inattention. Minimal involuntary movements.

4 Mild abnormality of tone or minimal or occasional associated reactions with effort. Can control tone but occasional abnormal tone, e.g., after activity. Purposeful accurate voluntary movement. Abnormal speed of movement. Minimal sensory inattention.

5 Normal purposeful skilled movement. Normal tone, normal sensory awareness, normal righting and equilibrium reactions, alert and orientated.

Disability

0 No purposeful active movement, totally dependent, requires full physical care and constant vigilant supervision. May have totally disruptive and uncooperative behavior. Dependent on skilled assistance.

1 Bed-chair-bound but unable to sit independently. Transfers with maximal assistance, wheelchair dependent, unable to stand unsupported. Some very limited purposeful activity. Needs high level of assistance in all tasks. Some awareness, some effort and recognition to contribute to care. Dependent on skilled assistance.

2 Head and trunk control. Limited self-help skills. Initiates some aspects of ADL. Transfers with one, mobilizes with two. Requires physical and/or verbal prompting and supervision for most tasks and movements. Participating in care and engaging in some structured activity. Dependent on skilled assistance.

3 Stands unsupported, transfers or walking requires supervision or help of one. "Household walker." Undertakes personal care in modified supported environment. Appropriately initiating activities and needs assistance or supervision with some unfamiliar or complex tasks. Initiates activities appropriately. Ability varies with time of day.

4   Carrying out personal care and tasks but is less efficient, clumsy, requires extra time or may need encouragement. Uses prompts effectively. Minimal or occasional assistance required for some complex tasks.

5   Age appropriate independence.

Handicap

0   Social isolation, no interaction, very little quality of life, no autonomy. Lack of self-esteem, or self-worth. Unable to exercise choice.

1   Very limited control of immediate environment, poor self-esteem, minimal autonomy with immediate carers only. Unable to exercise choice.

2   Marked loss or change of role, e.g., nonintegrated recreation, nonintegrated education/occupation, limited access to different community environments, autonomy in immediate environment. Limited choices available.

3   Has a role in some surroundings but this may be diminished or changed, e.g., unable to fulfill usual work or sport activities. Some limited access to general environment facilities, has autonomy within domicile and other familiar environments but limited choice and control in number of situations.

4   Some difficulty with sustaining expected roles (work, family, leisure), occasional restricted access to activities, reduced option for lifestyle. Has reduced choice and control in some situations.

5   Integrated and able to maintain expected different roles in society. Valued by others. Exercises choice and autonomy.

Distress/Well-Being

0   High and constant levels of concern/anger/severe depression or apathy, unable to express or control emotions appropriately.

1   Moderate concern, becomes concerned easily, requires constant reassurance/support, needs clear/tight limits and structure, loses emotional control easily.

2   Concern in unfamiliar situations, frequent emotional encouragement and support required.

3   Controls emotions with assistance, emotionally dependent on some occasions, vulnerable to change in routine, etc., spontaneously uses methods to assist emotional control.

4   Able to control feelings in most situations, generally well adjusted/stable (most of the time/most situations), occasional emotional support/encouragement needed.

5   Well adjusted, stable, and able to cope emotionally with most situations, good insight, accepts and understands own limitations.

RESPIRATORY CARE

Impairment

0 Full ventilatory support.

1 Some ventilatory support required, e.g., nighttime. Retains secretions/airway obstruction or altered air blood gases.

2 Requires regular oxygen therapy/medication. Altered use of respiratory muscles. Help required to clear secretions. Altered air blood gases.

3 Lung function maintained with regular medication. Frequently normal air blood gases. Frequent productive cough, occasional problem with self-clearing of secretions.

4 Normal lung function maintained with minimum medication. Nonproblematic self-clearing of secretions. Normal air blood gases.

5 Normal lung function.

Disability

0 Unable to move, breathlessness at rest. Total care required.

1 Severe breathlessness on movement in bed, severe orthopnea, breathlessness affecting fluency of speech, requires maximal help in all activities.

2 Severe breathlessness on minimal exertion, i.e., transfer from bed to chair, any effort affects speech, can undertake a few ADL tasks unaided.

3 Breathlessness on walking on level ground—50 yards. Normal speech when undertaking light activity. Independent for limited activities.

4 Breathlessness on flight of stairs, not breathless on level ground. Occasional activities restricted.

5 No functional disability, able to tackle exertion appropriate to age without respiratory distress.

Handicap

0 Social isolation, no interaction, very little quality of life, no autonomy. Lack of self-esteem, or self-worth. Unable to exercise choice.

1 Very limited control of immediate environment, poor self-esteem, minimal autonomy with immediate carers only. Unable to exercise choice.

2 Marked loss or change of role, e.g., nonintegrated recreation, nonintegrated education/occupation, limited access to different community environments, autonomy in immediate environment. Limited choices available.

3 Has a role in some surroundings but this may be diminished or changed, e.g., unable to fulfill usual work or sport activities. Some limited access to general environment facilities, has autonomy within domicile and other familiar environments but limited choice and control in number of situations.

4 Some difficulty with sustaining expected roles (work, family, leisure), occasional restricted access to activities, reduced option for lifestyle. Has reduced choice and control in some situations.

5 Integrated and able to maintain expected different roles in society. Valued by others. Exercises choice and autonomy.

Distress/Well-Being

0 High and constant levels of concern/anger/severe depression or apathy, unable to express or control emotions appropriately.

1 Moderate concern, becomes concerned easily, requires constant reassurance/support, needs clear/tight limits and structure, loses emotional control easily.

2 Concern in unfamiliar situations, frequent emotional encouragement and support required.

3 Controls emotions with assistance, emotionally dependent on some occasions, vulnerable to change in routine, etc., spontaneously uses methods to assist emotional control.

4 Able to control feelings in most situations, generally well adjusted/stable (most of the time/most situations), occasional emotional support/encouragement needed.

5 Well adjusted, stable, and able to cope emotionally with most situations, good insight, accepts and understands own limitations.

SCHIZOPHRENIA

Impairment

0   No insight, no volition, persistent/severe and wide range of thought disorder, fixed delusions, persistent visual, auditory, tactile hallucinations, persistent/severe disturbance of affect. Severe emotional blunting. Absence of empathy.

1   Thought disorder with variability, auditory hallucinations frequent, variable disturbance of affect, very little volition. Severe-moderate emotional blunting. Very occasional empathy present.

2   Moderate thought disorder in duration, severity, frequency, some auditory hallucinations present, moderate disturbance of affect, moderate level of volition. Moderate emotional blunting. Empathy present to a limited extent.

3   Occasional evidence of thought disorder in duration, severity, frequency, very occasional evidence of auditory hallucination, usually stable mood, volition intact. Occasional/mild emotional blunting. Appropriate empathy on occasions.

4   Very occasional evidence of some thought disorder in duration, severity, frequency, good level insight, usually stable mood, volition intact. No emotional blunting, appropriate empathy.

5   Well developed insight, high level of volition, no evidence of thought disorder, delusion, hallucinations, consistently stable mood.

Disability

0   Physically dependent for all functional tasks, bed-chair-bound, no self-care skills, inability to communicate, no attention.

1   Dependent for most tasks but will cooperate/assist with maximal prompting, needs cues and reminders for activities of daily living, occasional small amount of verbal communication with individual members of staff. No insight.

2   Able to initiate some aspects of activities of daily living, e.g., dressing. Understandable communication increased with some meaningful content, able to concentrate for a short time, easily distracted. Needs frequent supervision and prompting. Occasional insight.

3   Some consistency in communication, e.g., interacting with staff/carers and other clients, able to initiate a broader range of activities of daily living, responding to demands of rehabilitation.

4   Minimal assistance needed in less familiar environments, communicating effectively with a wide range of groups and individuals, concentrating on a majority of necessary activities. Uses self-help prompts well. Good insight.

5 Independent, no assistance needed for ADL, communicating effectively with a wide range of groups and individuals, concentrates on all necessary activities.

Handicap

0 Social isolation, no interaction, very little quality of life, no autonomy. Lack of self-esteem or self-worth. Unable to exercise choice.

1 Very limited control of immediate environment, poor self-esteem, minimal autonomy with immediate carers only. Unable to exercise choice.

2 Marked loss or change of role, e.g., nonintegrated recreation, nonintegrated education/occupation, limited access to different community environments, autonomy in immediate environment. Limited choices available.

3 Has a role in some surroundings but this may be diminished or changed, e.g., unable to fulfill usual work or sport activities. Some limited access to general environment facilities, has autonomy within domicile and other familiar environments but limited choice and control in number of situations.

4 Some difficulty with sustaining expected roles (work, family, leisure), occasional restricted access to activities, reduced option for lifestyle. Has reduced choice and control in some situations.

5 Integrated and able to maintain expected different roles in society. Valued by others. Exercises choice and autonomy.

Distress/Well-Being

0 High and constant levels of concern/anger/severe depression or apathy, unable to express or control emotions appropriately.

1 Moderate concern, becomes concerned easily, requires constant reassurance/support, needs clear/tight limits and structure, loses emotional control easily.

2 Concern in unfamiliar situations, frequent emotional encouragement and support required.

3 Controls emotions with assistance, emotionally dependent on some occasions, vulnerable to change in routine, etc., spontaneously uses methods to assist emotional control.

4 Able to control feelings in most situations, generally well adjusted/stable (most of the time/most situations), occasional emotional support/encouragement needed.

5 Well adjusted, stable, and able to cope emotionally with most situations, good insight, accepts and understands own limitations.

STROKE

Impairment

0   No voluntary movement, severe flaccidity or spasticity (Oxford Scale 0 for affected side), gross sensory impairment, loss of bowel and bladder control. Unresponsive.

1   Severe degree of several signs and symptoms, e.g., dense hemiplegia (Oxford Scale 1), severe perceptual deficit, occasional control of bladder and bowel, severe cognitive deficit, strong associated reactions with very limited range of passive movements. Responsive.

2   Moderate degree of several signs and symptoms, e.g., moderate hemiplegia and some dyspraxia (Oxford Scale 2), may have some bowel/bladder dysfunction. Active movement with gravity eliminated, control patterns of movement, moderate associated reactions, severe to moderate sensory deficit.

3   Active movement against gravity, controlled isolated movement, occasional associated reactions, moderate sensory inattention, movements may not be accurate, or one severe sign/symptom, e.g., dense hemiplegic arm, or two moderate signs/symptoms, e.g., moderate arm/leg hemiplegia (Oxford Scale 3).

4   Loss of fine active movement and coordination, minimal sensory deficit, loss of end range of movement. Slight incoordination or loss of power in limb/s, occasional perceptual cognitive or perceptual difficulties (Oxford Scale 4).

5   No impairment.

Disability

0   No purposeful active movement, totally dependent, requires full physical care and constant vigilant supervision. May have totally disruptive and uncooperative behavior. Dependent on skilled assistance.

1   Bed-chair-bound but unable to sit independently. Some very limited purposeful activity. Needs high level of assistance in most tasks. Some awareness, some effort and recognition to contribute to care. Dependent on skilled assistance.

2   Head and trunk control. Limited self-help skills. Initiates some aspects of ADL. Transfers with one, mobilizes with two. Requires physical and verbal prompting and supervision for most tasks and movements. Participating in care and engaging in some structured activity. Dependent on skilled assistance.

3   Transfers or walking requires supervision or help of one. Undertakes personal care in modified supported environment. Needs assistance or supervision with some unfamiliar or complex tasks. Initiates activities appropriately.

4   Carrying out personal care and tasks but is less efficient, clumsy, requires extra time or may need encouragement. Uses memory prompts effectively. Minimal or occasional assistance required for some complex tasks.

5 Age appropriate independence.

Handicap

0 Social isolation, no interaction, very little quality of life, no autonomy. Lack of self-esteem or self-worth. Unable to exercise choice.

1 Very limited control of immediate environment, poor self-esteem, minimal autonomy with immediate carers only. Unable to exercise choice.

2 Marked loss or change of role, e.g., nonintegrated recreation, nonintegrated education/occupation, limited access to different community environments, autonomy in immediate environment. Limited choices available.

3 Has a role in some surroundings but this may be diminished or changed, e.g., unable to fulfill usual work or sport activities. Some limited access to general environment facilities, has autonomy within domicile and other familiar environments but limited choice and control in number of situations.

4 Some difficulty with sustaining expected roles (work, family, leisure), occasional restricted access to activities, reduced option for lifestyle. Has reduced choice and control in some situations.

5 Integrated and able to maintain expected different roles in society. Valued by others. Exercises choice and autonomy.

Distress/Well-Being

0 High and constant levels of concern/anger/severe depression or apathy, unable to express or control emotions appropriately.

1 Moderate concern, becomes concerned easily, requires constant reassurance/support, needs clear/tight limits and structure, loses emotional control easily.

2 Concern in unfamiliar situations, frequent emotional encouragement and support required.

3 Controls emotions with assistance, emotionally dependent on some occasions, vulnerable to change in routine, etc., spontaneously uses methods to assist emotional control.

4 Able to control feelings in most situations, generally well adjusted/stable (most of the time/most situations), occasional emotional support/encouragement needed.

5 Well adjusted, stable and able to cope emotionally with most situations, good insight, accepts and understands own limitations.

WOUND CARE

Impairment

0   Black/necrotic full thickness wound or large surface area wound, e.g., burn or large fungating wound with involvement of major blood vessels. Severe continual pain.

1   Deep wound extending to muscle, infected and inflamed or medium surface area wound. Severe pain, some relief with medication.

2   Sloughy wound, subcutaneous damage. Medium exudate, offensive smell. Moderate pain or occasional severe pain, relieved with medication.

3   Granulating clean wound. Epidermal damage, blistered, moist. Pain well controlled.

4   Superficial skin break. Inflamed, reddened area. Occasional discomfort.

5   Skin intact, healthy and pink

Disability

0   Bed-bound, semiconscious. Totally dependent.

1   Bed-chair-bound, requires maximum assistance with tasks but cooperates.

2   Chair-bound, limited mobility, requires frequent assistance of one person. Can undertake some tasks independently.

3   Mobile with minimum assistance/supervision, requires some nursing intervention.

4   Can live independently. Mainly self-caring with occasional monitoring by others.

5   Totally independent and able to function normally.

Handicap

0   Social isolation, no interaction, very little quality of life, no autonomy. Lack of self-esteem or self-worth. Unable to exercise choice.

1   Very limited control of immediate environment, poor self-esteem, minimal autonomy with immediate carers only. Unable to exercise choice.

2   Marked loss or change of role, e.g., nonintegrated recreation, nonintegrated education, limited access to different community environments, autonomy immediate in environment. Limited choices available.

3   Has a role in some surroundings but this may be diminished or changed, e.g., unable to fulfill usual work or sport activities. Some limited access to general environment facilities, has autonomy within domicile and other familiar environments but limited choice and control in number of situations.

4   Some difficulty with sustaining expected roles (work, family, leisure), occasional restricted access to activities, reduced option for lifestyle. Has reduced choice and control in some situations.

5   Integrated and able to maintain expected roles in society. Valued by others. Exercises choice and autonomy.

Distress/Well-Being

0   Severe constant anxiety/depression, unable to express emotions appropriately.

1   Severe anxiety/frequent bouts of depression. Severe frustration.

2   Moderate anxiety/regular bouts of depression. Positive responses after reinforcement.

3   Moderate anxiety/occasional bouts of depression. Showing initiative, responsible.

4   Mild anxiety/occasional controllable depression. Well adjusted.

5   No distress, well adjusted.

Appendix 3

Physiotherapist/Occupational Therapist Etiologies and Disorders

Etiology Codes

1. Respiratory Disease
   a. Chronic
   b. Acute
   c. Other
2. Obs. & Gyne. Disorders
   a. Incontinence
   b. Other
3. Spinal Disorders
   a. Spinal Surgery
   b. Low Back Pain
   c. Thoracic Pain
   d. Cervical Pain
   e. Other
4. Musculoskeletal
   a. J.C.A.
   b. Osteoarthritis
   c. Soft Tissue Injuries
   d. Joint Problems
   e. Rheumatoid Arthritis
   f. Other
5. Orthopedic
   a. Fracture/Dislocation
   b. Joint Replacement
   c. Spinal Injury
   d. Other
6. Amputations
7. Mental Illness
   a. Addictions
   b. Forensic
   c. Functional EMI
   d. Organic EMI
   e. Schizophrenia/Affective Disorders
   f. Other
8. Cardiovascular Disease
   a. M.I.
   b. Thrombosis
   c. Other
9. Acquired Neurological
   a. Guillan Barré
   b. C.V.A.
   c. Head Injury
   d. Dementia
   e. Other
10. Peripheral Neuropathy
11. Neurosurgery (Brain)
12. Surgery
    a. General
    b. Cardiothoracic
13. Progressive Neurological Disease
    a. M.S.
    b. P.D.
    c. M.N.D.
    d. Muscular Dystrophy
    e. Other
14. Dermatology
15. Burns/Plastics
16. Congenital Neurological
    a. C.P.
    b. Dyspraxia
    c. Other
17. Learning Difficulties
18. Multifactorial
19. Nothing Abnormal Detected
20. Other (please specify)

Physiotherapy/OT Disorders

1. Abnormal Joint Mobility
   a. Abnormal Muscle Length
   b. Other
2. Inadequate Muscle Power
3. Abnormal Muscle Tone
4. Delayed or Abnormal Development
5. Coordination Problems
6. Altered Circulation
7. Pain
8. Sensory/Perceptual impairment
9. Prevention Complications
10. Abnormal Cardiac Function
11. Abnormal Respiratory Function
12. Behavioral/Psychosocial
13. Multifactorial Problems
    a. Multisystem Failure
    b. Neurological
    c. Profound Multiple Difficulties
    d. Other
14. Decreased General Mobility
15. Nothing Abnormal Detected
16. Other (please specify)

Appendix 4

OUTCOME MEASURES
CLIENT DETAILS

Patient Name or Identifying Code Number

Therapy Profession _____
(Speech, Physiotherapy, Nursing, Diet, O.T.)

NHS District/Trust _____

Patient Details

Age _____
(Years)

Duration of Treatment _____
(Months)

No. of Contacts _____

Locality
Tick appropriate box

☐ Inpatient

☐ Outpatient

☐ Community

Carer _____
(Spouse, Mother, etc.)

Client Care Group
Tick appropriate box

☐ Child

☐ Adult

Etiology Code
(see overleaf for codes)

[   ] [   ]

Disorder Code 1
(See overleaf for codes)

[   ] [   ]

Disorder Code 2
(as above)

[   ] [   ]

Ratings

Code*	Impairment Imp1	Imp2	Disability	Handicap	Well-being Patient	Carer	Agreement	Date
A							NA	/ /
								/ /
								/ /
								/ /
								/ /
								/ /

* A = Admission, I = Intermediate, F = Final.

Comments _____

_____

Appendix 5

OUTCOME MEASURES
SAMPLE CLIENT DETAILS

1 | Patient Name or Identifying Code Number
JAMES BOND 007

2 Therapy Profession ___*PHYSIOTHERAPY*___
(Speech, Physiotherapy, Nursing, Diet, O.T.)

3 NHS District/Trust ___*ST ELSEWHERES*___

Patient Details

4
Age ___*39*___
(Years)

5
Duration of Treatment ___*6*___
(Months)

6
No. of Contacts ___*21*___

7
Locality
Tick appropriate box

☐ Inpatient

☑ Outpatient

☐ Community

8
Carer ___*SPOUSE*___
(Spouse, Mother, etc.)

9
Client Care Group
Tick appropriate box

☐ Child

☑ Adult

10
Etiology Code
(see overleaf for codes)

[3] [C]

11
Disorder Code 1
(See overleaf for codes)

[4] [   ]

Disorder Code 2
(as above)

[6] [   ]

Ratings

Code*	(13) Impairment		Disability	Handicap	Well-being		Agreement	Date
	Imp1	Imp2			Patient	Carer		
A	1	3	2	3	3	2	NA	12/06/95
I	3	3	35	4	4	3	2	06/09/95
F	35	3	4	4	4	4	3	08/12/95
								/ /
								/ /
								/ /

* A = Admission, I = Intermediate, F = Final.

14
Comments _____

_____

Appendix 6

OUTCOME MEASURES DATA FORM GUIDANCE NOTES

1. **Patient's name or identifying code number**
   This information is not to be stored on computer.

2. **Therapy Profession**
   Please detail which therapy profession you belong to. Date will be analyzed by profession.

3. **NHS District/Trust**
   Please identify the Authority/Trust for which you work.

4. **Age**
   Please detail the age of the patient when you recorded their admission score (see point 9 below). Record years, or fraction of years for young children.

5. **Duration of Treatment**
   Detail the duration of treatment in months.

6. **Number of Contacts**
   Detail the amount of attention you have given to a patient. These may be attendances or time spent in influencing care, e.g., discussions with family, etc. A rough guide to your involvement is all that is needed, e.g., 2 attendances + 1 chat with relatives + 1 chat with nurse in charge = 4.

7. **Locality**
   Please tick the area in which the patient is treated. You can tick more than one of these boxes if the patient's locality changes during the recorded treatment period.

8. **Carer**
   Please detail the person (if any) who was involved in defining the agreement score, i.e., anybody else other than the patient themselves.

9. **Client Care Group**
   Identify whether the client is being seen as part of child or adult services by ticking the box.

10. **Etiology & Impairment Codes**
    Select the code from code sheet. If client has more than one impairment, identify the most relevant to episode of care first.

11. **Ratings**
    A **Admission.** Detail the Outcome Score of the patient when you are first starting treatment. This row of scores will not have an agreement rating.
    I **Intermediate.** If you alter treatment or have ended an episode of care but without discharging the patient, gauge an Outcome Score and code appropriately, you can have several "I" scores. Record an agreement rating.
    F **Final.** Rate the ultimate outcome at discharge from the therapy session/service. Record an agreement rating as above.

12. Select the score most closely representing your patient's ability. Remember they do not have to be exactly as the descriptor suggests. The descriptors are to help gauge the relative degrees of ISIDHWCW.* Half points (e.g., 2.5) indicate if you think a person is slightly better or worse than a particular score point. If the client has two impairments rate both but rate both but rate the one most relevant to episode of care first.

13. **Well-Being Score**
    Well-being of the client is reflected in the left hand space. Well-being of the carer (if relevant) is reflected in the right hand space.

14. **Comment**
    Please use this section to indicate to the Researchers any concerns that you have with the Outcome Scores not reflecting or being difficult to reflect for that individual patient.

---

1 Patient Name or Identifying Code Number

JAMES BOND 007

2 Therapy Profession   PHYSIOTHERAPY
(Speech, Physiotherapy, Nursing, Diet, O.T.)

3 NHS District/Trust   ST ELSEWHERES

Patient Details

4 Age 39 (Years)

5 Duration of Treatment 6 (Months)

6 No. of Contacts 21

7 Locality
Tick appropriate box

☐ Inpatient

☑ Outpatient

☐ Community

8 Carer SPOUSE (Spouse, Mother, etc.)

9 Client Care Group
Tick appropriate box

☐ Child

☑ Adult

10 Etiology Code
(see overleaf for codes)

[3] [C]

11 Disorder Code 1
(See overleaf for codes)

[4] [ ]

Disorder Code 2
(as above)

[6] [ ]

Ratings

Code*	(13) Impairment Imp1	Imp2	Disability	Handicap	Well-being Patient	Carer	Agreement	Date
A	1	3	2	3	3	2	N/A	12/06/95
I	3	3	35	4	4	3	2	06/09/95
F	35	3	4	4	4	4	3	08/12/95
								/ /
								/ /
								/ /

* A = Admission, I = Intermediate, F = Final.

14 Comments _____

---

* **I** - Impairment, **SI** - Second Impairment, **D** - Disability, **H** - Handicap, **W** - Well-being, **CW** - Carer's Well-being.

Appendix 7

Core Scales:
Learning Prompt Sheet

Impairment

Each team member should rate the severity of the presentation of the disorder as it affects the person's/child's capacities (*for their age*) in their specific area (e.g., gross motor skills, physical deficit, communication, cognition, psychological disorder).

Very severe	Severe	Severe/ Moderate	Moderate	Mild	No Impairment
0 / 0.5	1 / 1.5	2 / 2.5	3 / 3.5	4 / 4.5	5

Disability/Activity

Each team member should rate the degree to which a person's/child's impairment affects his/her ability to perform a task/function/interact *at an age-appropriate level* (e.g., mobility, dexterity, communication of needs, self-feeding, learning, independence, appropriateness of emotional responses, behavior).

Unable to perform task/ totally dependent on others/no awareness of surroundings	Assists/ cooperates but burden of task falls on carers/ some awareness of surroundings	Can undertake some part of task but needs a high level of support to complete/some interaction with environment	Can undertake task/function/ interaction in familiar situation but needs verbal/ physical assistance at other times	Requires some minor assistance occasionally or extra time to complete task	Age- appropriately/ independent/ able to function/ perform task/ interacts with environment appropriately
0 / 0.5	1 / 1.5	2 / 2.5	3 / 3.5	4 / 4.5	5

Handicap/Participation

The whole team should rate the degree to which a person's/child's impairment affects his/her (age related) functioning within a social context/the family, i.e., ability to make choices and have control over lives/environment; self-awareness and confidence; integration into age-appropriate activities; achievement of potential. This dimension reflects the capabilities of the patient as well as the environment and those in the environment.

Isolated, no control over environment, no relationships, unable to exercise choice "too protected"/	Very limited choices, little control over life, some awareness of self within environment, very abnormal role/control	Able to make some choices, able to access nonintegrated facilities, moderately abnormal role in family/ environment	Some supported integration, achievement of potential with encouragement, some control over life, some abnormal control/role	Mostly confident, occasionally some restriction in integration or lack of confidence	Integrated, valued, and autonomous in family and society
0 / 0.5	1 / 1.5	2 / 2.5	3 / 3.5	4 / 4.5	5

Well-Being/Distress

The team should rate the degree of upset affecting the child and parents/carers (2 scores) *

Severe consistent distress, complete detachment no appropriate emotions	Severe consistent distress frequently experienced; mainly detached	Moderate consistent distress, severe occasional distress, frequent detachment	Moderate distress frequently experienced, often inappropriately detached	Distress occasionally experienced, occasional inappropriate detachment	No inappropriate distress/ detachment
0 / 0.5	1 / 1.5	2 / 2.5	3 / 3.5	4 / 4.5	5

* Do not try to attribute distress to any aspect of the person's life or difficulties. Rate this overall even if you think the degree of upset is related to some extraneous issue, e.g., finances/housing.